LIFE SCIENCE
in
TOOLS & TECHNIQUES

LIFE SCIENCE in TOOLS & TECHNIQUES

By

P.S. BISEN
D.Sc.
Department of Microbiology
Barkatullah University
Bhopal 462 026

SHRUTI MATHUR
M.Sc.
Department of Microbiology
Barkatullah University
Bhopal 462 026

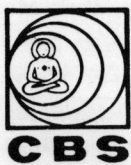

C B S

CBS Publishers & Distributors Pvt. Ltd.

New Delhi • Bengaluru • Chennai • Kochi • Kolkata • Mumbai
Hyderabad • Nagpur • Patna • Pune • Vijayawada

ISBN: 81-239-0318-9

First Edition: 1998
Reprint: 2004, 2006, 2009, 2016

Published by:
Satish Kumar Jain for CBS Publishers & Distributors Pvt. Ltd.,
4819/XI Prahlad Street, 24 Ansari Road, Daryaganj, New Delhi - 110002
delhi@cbspd.com, cbspubs@airtelmail.in • www.cbspd.com
Ph.: 23289259, 23266861, 23266867 • Fax: 011-23243014

Corporate Office: 204 FIE, Industrial Area, Patparganj, Delhi - 110 092
Ph: 49344934 • Fax: 011-49344935
E-mail: publishing@cbspd.com • publicity@cbspd.com

Branches:
• *Bengaluru:* 2975, 17th Cross, K.R. Road, Bansankari 2nd Stage,
  Bengaluru - 70 • Ph: +91-80-26771678/79 • Fax: +91-80-26771680
  E-mail: cbsbng@gmail.com, bangalore@cbspd.com
• *Chennai:* No. 7, Subbaraya Street, Shenoy Nagar, Chennai - 600030
  Ph: +91-44-26681266, 26680620 • Fax: +91-44-42032115
  E-mail: chennai@cbspd.com
• *Kochi:* Ashana House, 39/1904, A.M. Thomas Road, Valanjambalam,
  Ernakulum, Kochi • Ph: +91-484-4059061-65
  Fax: +91-484-4059065 • E-mail: cochin@cbspd.com
• *Kolkata:* 6-B, Ground Floor, Rameshwar Shaw Road, Kolkata - 700014
  Ph: +91-33-22891126/7/8 • E-mail: kolkata@cbspd.com
• *Mumbai:* 83-C, Dr. E. Moses Road, Worli, Mumbai - 400018
  Ph: +91-9833017933, 022-24902340/41 • E-mail: mumbai@cbspd.com

Representatives:

• Hyderabad: 0-9885175004	• Nagpur: 0-9021734563
• Patna: 0-9334159340	• Pune: 0-9623451994
• Vijayawada: 0-9000660880	

Printed at:
J.S. Offset Printers, Delhi

PREFACE

The current technological boom has put forth a variety of techniques being used in scientific research. There is now, more than ever, a great deal of interaction between the physical and biological sciences. The biologist today depends on instrumentation to study the physiology and genetics of living organisms, particularly so at the molecular level. There is, therefore, a need for thorough understanding of the physical principles involved in operation of instruments and the parameters of study required in using the instrument. This book is an endeavour towards that end.

Chapter 1 deals with microscopy. The microscope began as a special arrangement of glass lenses. Today, different illumination methods and the use of electromagnetic lenses has given rise to a variety of different types of more specialised microscopes having better resolution; all of which has been explained in considerable detail in the chapter.

Chapter 2 deals with chromatography. Based on a simple physical rule of partition equilibrium, it creates a variety of very sensitive instruments when interfaced with other materials like solids and gases in a special arrangement of apparatus.

Chapter 3 throws light on spectroscopy. This technique uses the different regions of the electromagnetic spectrum to excite molecules and obtain information on their structure based on absorbance and emission characteristics.

Chapter 4 deals with how centrifugal force could be put to use not only for preparative but also for analytical purposes.

Chapter 5 is an insight in manometeric techniques used to measure gas exchanges in living cells.

Chapter 6 focusses on electrophoretic techniques and their applications to study the molecular nature of cell components.

X-Ray Microanalysis was initially used exclusively for physical and applied sciences particularly in metallurgy. Of late, it has become possible to study living materials also using this technique. Chapter 7 explains the principles involved in the process.

Chapter 8 deals with principles involved in using such common place instruments as the pH meter and the not so common oxygen-electrode. Both, extremely useful in the laboratory.

What was an accidental discovery for Madam Curie is today an indispensable tool in Life Sciences. Radioactivity is the ultimate in research at the molecular level. Chapter 9 deals extensively on the applications of this phenomenon in biology.

The all pervading Personal Computer has been programmed to analyse and organise bulky data and arrive at intelligible results. The last chapter introduces this and other aspects of the PC.

All chapters have been organised from the basic to the practical with appropriate illustrations to make them comprehensive.

The book would be useful for undergraduate and post-graduate students of Life Science as an introduction to the tools and techniques concurrently in practice. The book can also help the researcher by laying down the list of methods and their principles which could be put to practice to further his study.

Suggestion and corrections are welcome for further editions.

AUTHORS

CONTENTS

MICROSCOPY

1. INTRODUCTION

A microscope is defined as an instrument magnifying objects by means of lenses so as to reveal details invisible to the naked eye.

Only after the discovery of the first microscope around 1590 by a dutch spectacle maker Zaccharias Jensen, it was realised that there were certain living organisms so small in size that they were invisible to the naked eye and hence never believed to be existing. The microscope therefore opened new doors into the living world bringing forth a realm of microorganisms. This gave concrete evidence to Louis Pasteur's germ theory of disease. Thus began the science of microbiology.

Through the microscope the different shapes sizes and even colours of microorganisms can be seen. The degree of magnification needed to see a microorganism depends upon the size of the microbe. Protozoa, fungi, algae, bacteria whose sizes range from 1-200 μm can be viewed with a light microscope i.e., a microscope that uses visible light to illuminate the specimen. It magnifies about 1500X. Smaller microorganisms like viruses whose size varies from 0.015-2 μm, as well as internal structure of bacterial cells or eukaryotic cell organelles require the use of more specialised electron microscope which has a higher magnification 200,000X (Table.1.1). It may be noted here that the extent of magnification is limited by the capacity of resolution which we shall discuss later. Without resolution, magnification is called empty magnification and is of practically no use whatsoever.

Table 1.1

Type of Microscope	Maximum useful magnification	Resolution	Useful Application
Bright field	1500 X	100-200nm	Extensively used for visualisation of microorganisms and their gross morphological features; usually staining is necessary to view specimens.

(Contd.)

Type of Microscope	Maximum useful magnification	Resolution	Useful Application
Dark field	1500 X	100-200 nm	Used for viewing live microorganisms particularly those with characteristic morphology eg. spirochaetes. Staining not required Specimen appears bright on a dark background.
Phase contrast	1500X	100-200 nm	Used to examine cellular structures of living cells of yeast algae, protozoa and some bacteria does not require staining.
Interference	1500X	100-200 nm	Used to examine structure of microorganisms, produces sharp, multicoloured image with 3-D appearance.
UV	2500X	100 nm	Useful for obtaining improved resolution, largely replaced by electron microscope.
Fluorescence	1500X	100-200 nm	Used for fluorescent staining. Useful in many diagnostic procedures for identifying microorganisms.
TEM	500,000 X 1000,000X	1 nm	Used to view ultrastructure of microorganisms including viruses, much greater resolving power and useful magnification achieved than with light microscope.
SEM	10,000X- 1000,000X	1-10 nm	Used for viewing surface structures in detail, produces a 3-D image.

Today, the microbiologist has a variety of microscopes at his disposal (Table. 1.1). Together with the different techniques available for exploration, he can choose and use them for study. The choice of a particular microscope depends on the size of the object, the degree of detail to be viewed and the purpose of microscopic observation.

In this chapter, we shall examine the different types of microscopes, their advantages and disadvantages and also analytical techniques using the microscope.

In order to understand the indispensable role played by the microscope in the study of microorganisms, it is necessary to appreciate the intrinsic limitation of the eye as a magnifying instrument. The image formed by the eyelens L (Fig. 1.1) must appear on the retina R, in order to be clearly seen. The ciliary muscles attached to the lens surfaces can alter the focal length of the lens. This enables the eye to focus different distances on the retina, a property of the eye known as it's power of accomodation. However, the eye cannot accomodate objects brought closer to it than approximately 25 cm due to muscular orientation.

1.1   Magnification, Resolution and Contrast.

In order to view an object closer to the eye than 25 cms, a converging lens is placed between the object (at less than 25 cms from the eye) and the eye. This produces an enlarged virtual image at 25 cms from the eye (Fig. 1.2). The apparent size of an object

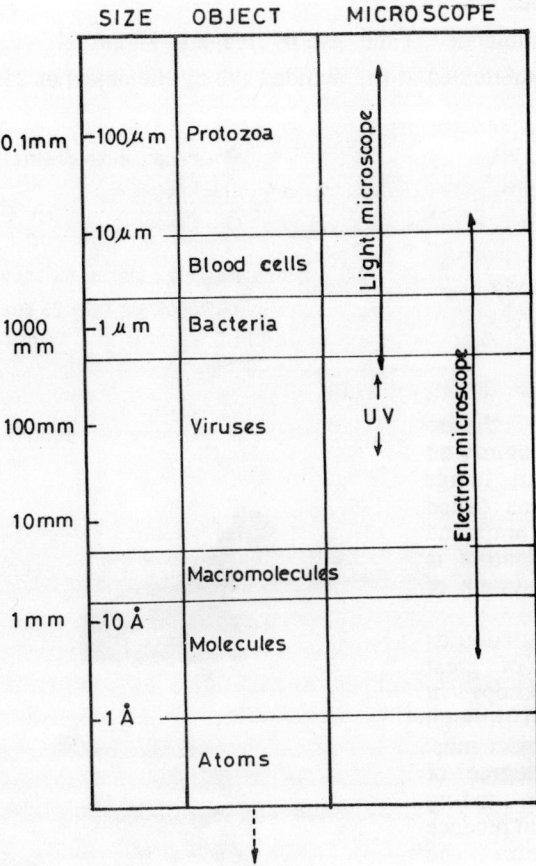

Table 1. Relative size of microbes, molecules, and atoms is depicted here together with an indication of the usefull range of different types of microscopes.

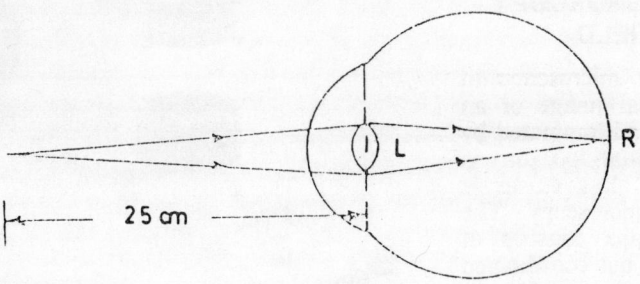

Fig. 1.1 : Image formation on the Retina of the eye.

as viewed by the unaided eye is directly related to the angle that the object subtends at the eye. Magnification is achieved by increasing the angle subtended by the image at the eye so that the size of the object apparently increases from h to h' (Fig. 1.2). Magnification is therefore defined as M = 0'/0 where, M = magnification

θ' = angle subtended at the eye by image at 25 cm

θ = angle subtended at the unaided eye by the object at 25 cm

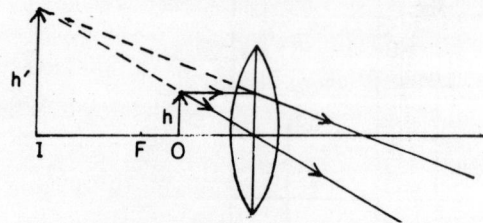

F = Focal length of lens,

I = Image,

O = Object.

Fig. 1.2 : Use of a converging lens to view an object closer than 25 cm to the eye.

The principle of a compound microscope is the use of an eye piece to magnify an already enlarged real image produced by a first lens called an objective. In a compound microscope magnification is brought about by a system of lenses.

Two other factors; contrast and resolution are of great importance in microscopy. In order to be perceived through the microscope an object must possess a certain degree of contrast with its surrounding medium and in order to produce useful magnification the microscpe must have resolution, that is, ability to discern two closely adjacent points as separate.

2. LIGHT MICROSCOPY - BRIGHT FIELD

The use of a microscope in which the final image of an object which is illuminated by visible light (400-700 μm) is seen through glass lenses is called light microscopy. The light microscope consists of three separate but coordinated lens sytems (Fig. 1.3). (i) condenser (ii) objective (iii) eye-piece. The total useful magnification produced is about 1500 X and is equal to the product of magnification of objective and eyepiece.

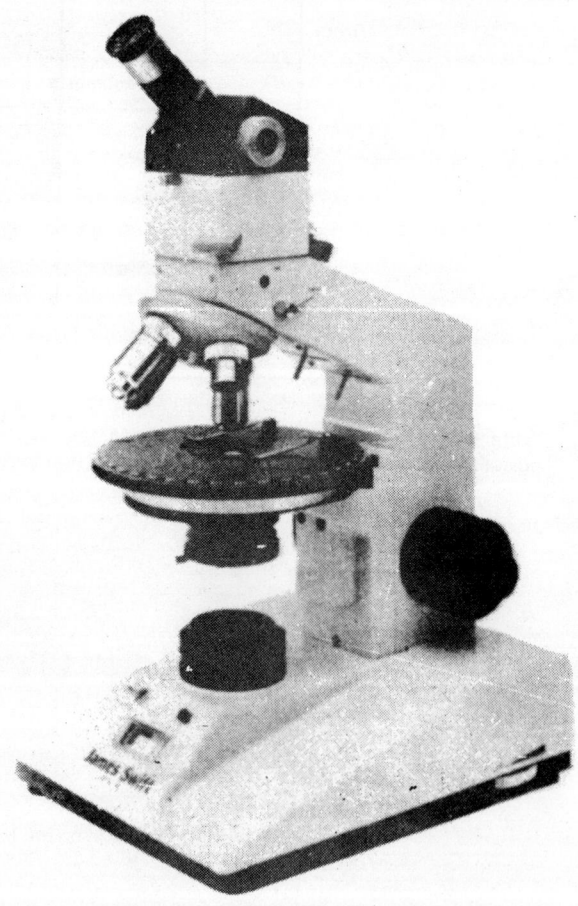

Fig. 1.3 (a) : The student microscope.

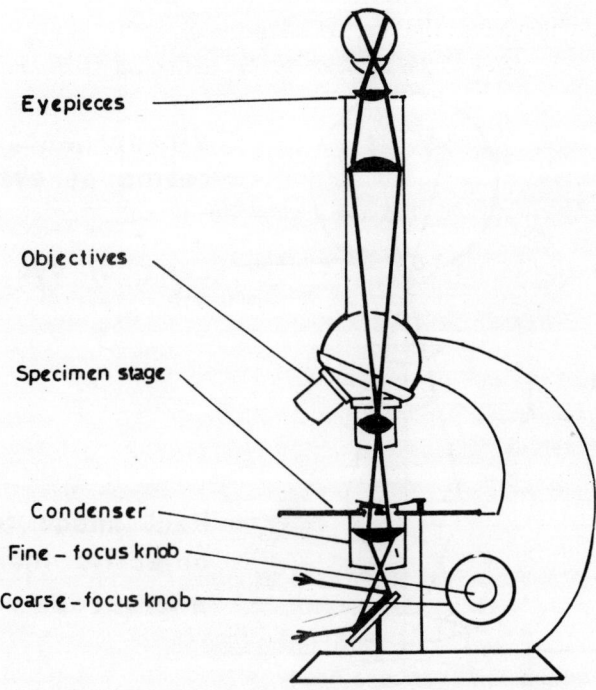

Fig. 1.3 (b) : Cutaway sketch of student microscope showing optical parts and path of light.

Condenser: Collimates light beam, regulates passage of light and eliminates peripheral rays from source. Occasionally there is also a sub stage condenser which concentrates light beam on the object. This effectively increases the numerical aperture, which, as will become clear later, increases the resolving power of the microscope.

Objective: The objective lens system magnifies about 90 X to 100 X and produces a real image inside the microscope.

Eyepiece: The eyepiece magnifies the real image to form a vertual image on the retina of the eye producing a total magnification of 1500 X. In the compound light microscope, light rays from below the condenser are refracted through the condenser and emerge from the top surface of the slide, at the plane of the object as a cone of light with the apex downward (Fig. 1.4).

Single lenses have two inherent defects :

1. Spherical Aberration
2. Chromatic Aberration

Spherical aberration is the inequalities of refraction and focus by the peripheral portions of the lens. This is due to the curved surface characteristics of the lens element. Rays at the outermost margins of the lens are refracted to a greater degree thereby forming the image at a point closer to the emergent side of the lens. This can be corrected either by combining with the lens, another lens of opposite diverging power or by using iris diaphragm which eliminates peripheral rays (Fig. 1.5 a).

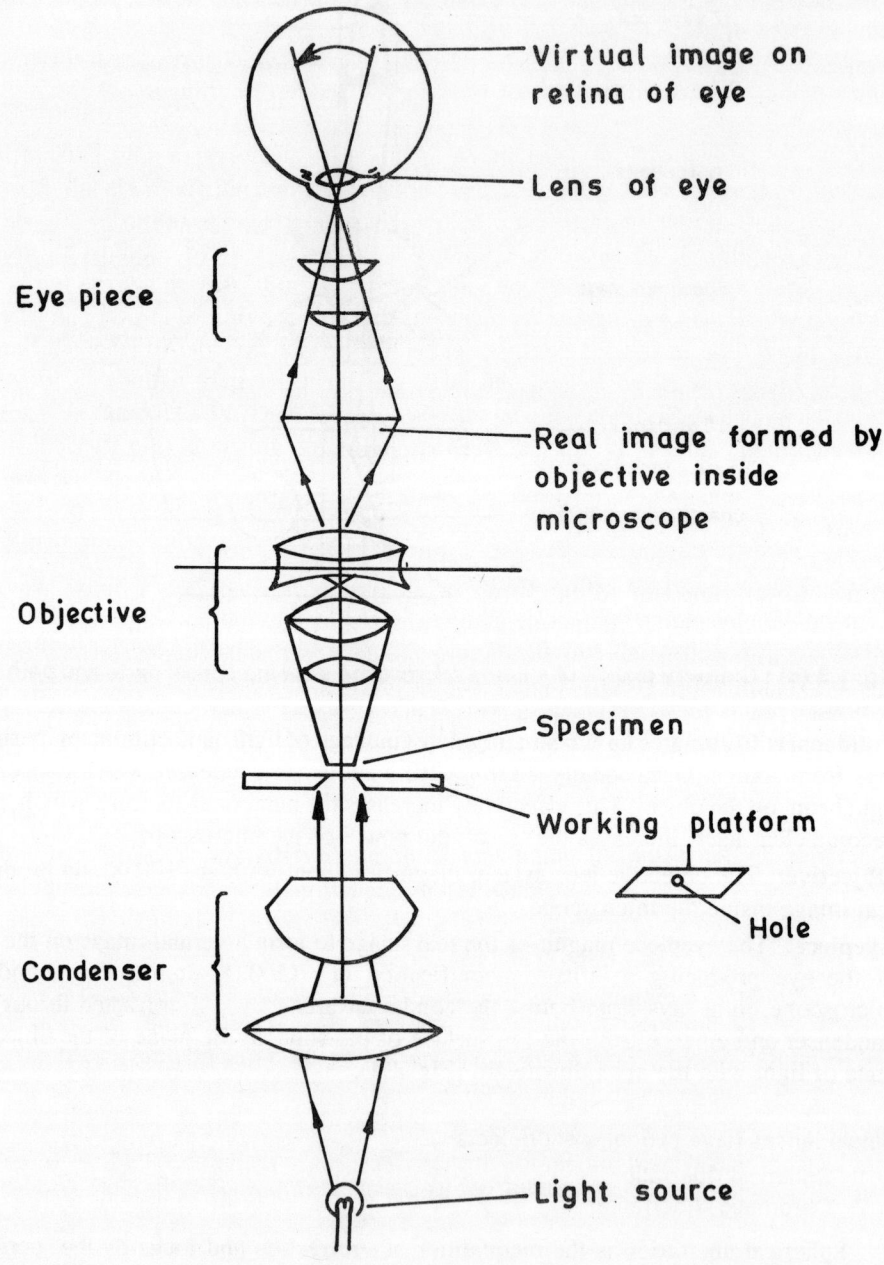

Fig. 1.4 Schematic Representation of Optical System of a Compound
Microscope

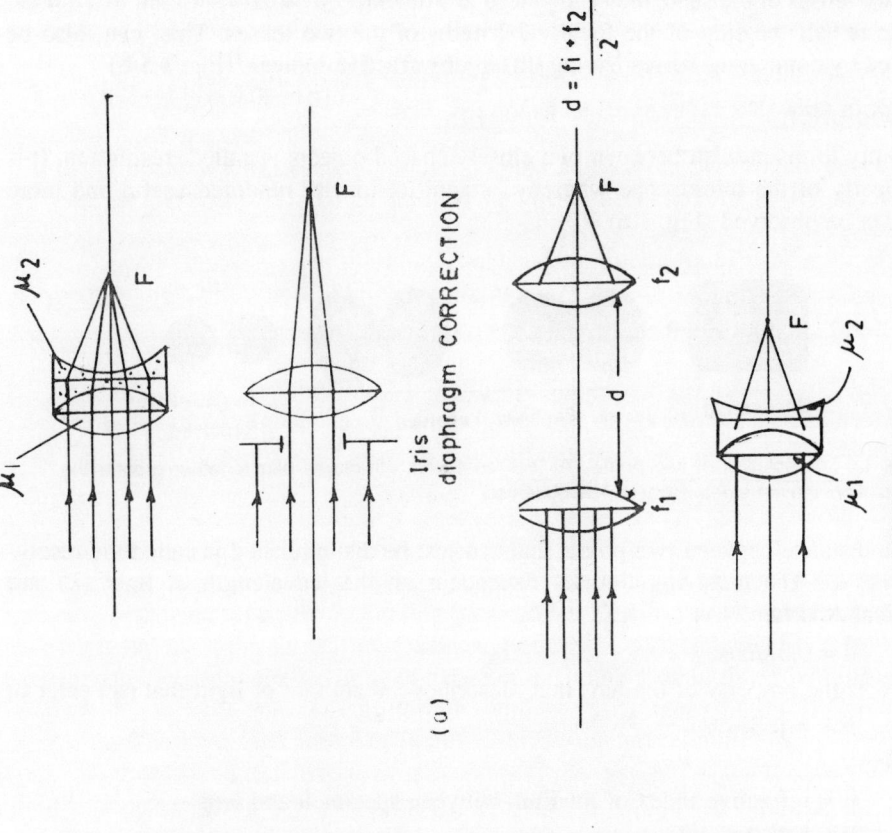

(a)

Iris
diaphragm CORRECTION

$$d = \frac{f_1 + f_2}{2}$$

(b)

CORRECTION

Fig. 1.5 : Lens defects and correction

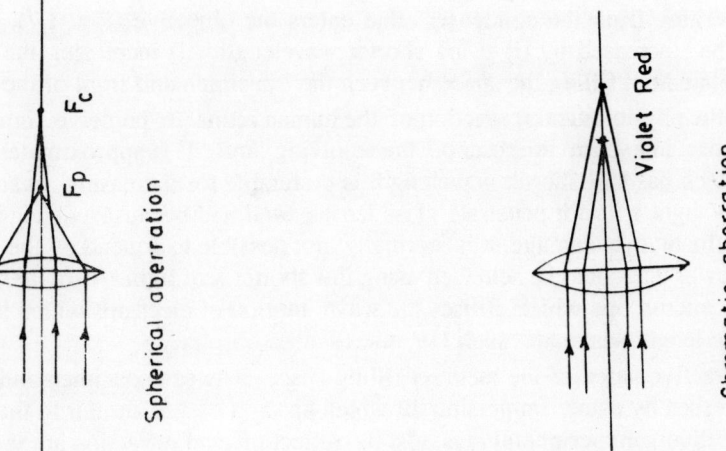

Spherical aberration

Chromatic aberration

Chromatic aberration is the inequalities of refraction and focus of all the different wavelengths of white light producing multiple coloured images. This is corrected by using two lenses of the same material placed at a distance 'd' apart such that $d = \frac{f + f}{2}$ i.e. distance is half the sum of the focal lengths of the two lenses. This can also be corrected by combining lenses having different refractive indices. (Fig. 1.5 b)

2.1 Resolution

The ability to distinguish between two closely spaced objects is called resolution. It is the property of the microscope whereby magnification is rendered useful and more detail can be observed (Fig. 1.6).

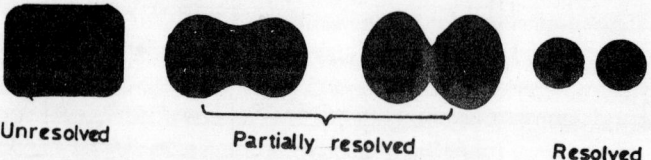

Fig. 1.6 : Resolution of two points. At low resolution, structures blur together greater the resolution, the more detail that can be observed.

The distance between two points that can just be distinguished is called the resolving limit 'd'. The resolving limit is dependent on the wavelength of light (λ) and Numerical Aperture(NA)

$$d = 0.5\lambda/NA$$

NA is the property of the lens that describes the amount of light that can enter it.

$$NA = \mu \, Sin \, \theta$$

Where,

μ = refractive index of medium between specimen and lens

θ = half the angular aperture

Angular aperture is the angle between the most divergent rays of the inverted cone of light emerging from the condenser that enters the objective (Fig. 1.7). Resolving power can be increased by (i) using shorter wavelength (ii) increasing the refractive index of the medium filling the space between the specimen and front of the objective.

Due to the physiological restriction of the human retina to perceive light between 400 to 700 nm, in a light microscope, the resolving limit 'd' is approximately 200 µm. UV light which has still shorter wavelength is preferable for increasing resolution but because UV light will not penetrate glass lenses well and because viewing UV light directly results in eye damage, it is normally not possible to depend on the improved resolving power that could be achieved using this shorter λ of light. Also, the advent of the electron microscope which utilises the wave motion of electrons which have much shorter wave length has made such UV microscopes obsolete.

The refractive index of the medium filling space between specimen and objective can be increased by using immersion oil which has a μ of 1.5, similar to that of glass. Many of the divergent peripheral rays lost by reflection and refraction at the surface of the condenser, slide and objective lens are refracted within the angular aperture thereby increasing the NA and consequently the resolution. It might be recalled that the use of

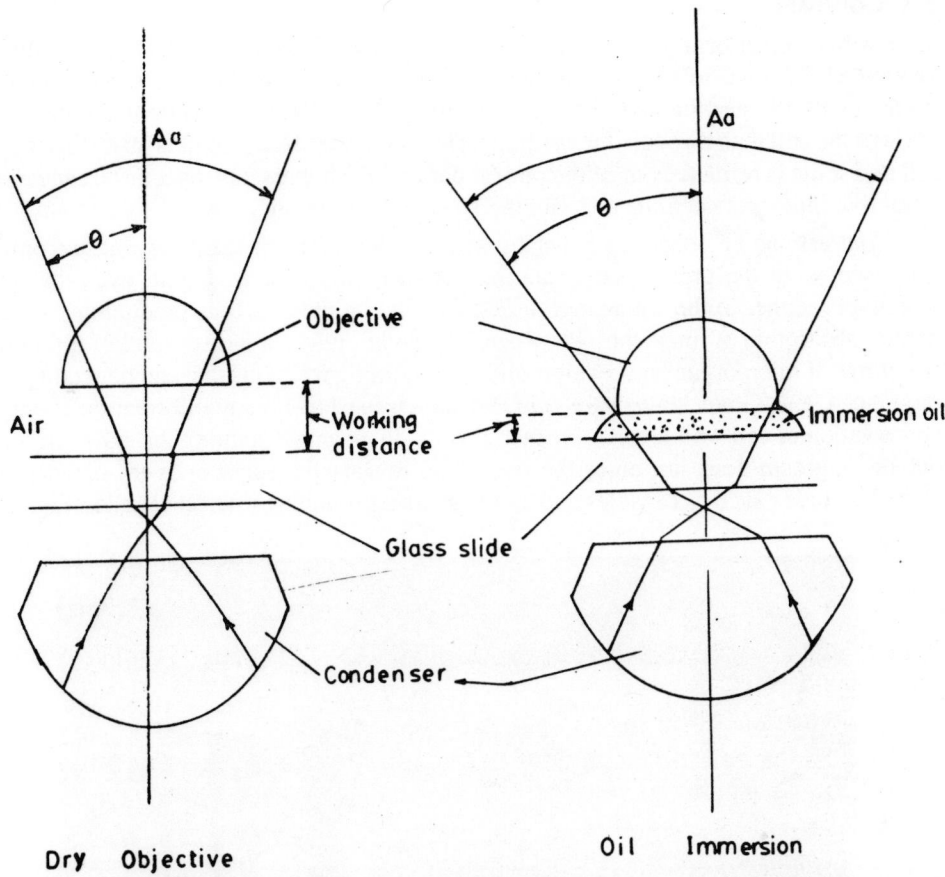

Dry   Objective   Oil   Immersion

Fig. 1.7 : The numercial aperture is improved by the use of immersion oil to replace the air between specimen on glass slide and objetive as shown by the wider angular aperture (Aa) Obtained using an oil immersion lens. * = Angle between the most divergent rays entering the objective and the optical axis and is equal to Half Aa. The working distance is also reduced in an oil immersion.

a substage condenser concentrates peripheral light waves on the object thereby, effectively increasing the NA, decreasing the resolving limit which means increasing the resolution.

Use of immersion oil also effectively decreases the focal length of the lens so that the specimen has to be very close to the objective in order to be focussed. Therefore there is a short working distance between lens and objective . A short focal length also reduces depth of field so that only very thin sections can be focussed.

The observation of algae, fungi and protozoa can be achieved with dry objectives, that is, when air occupies the space between specimen and objective. The viewing of bacteria which are smaller in size normally requires the use of oil immersion lens. Such lenses are specially designed for use with immersion oil and should never be used without it.

2.2 Contrast

A microbial cell is largely composed of water as is the medium in which it is normally suspended. In order to be seen through the microscope it should have some degree of contrast with the surrounding medium,the contrast arises because less light is transmitted through the cell than through the medium. This is because some light is absorbed by the cell and some is refracted out of the optical path of the microscope by a difference in the refractive index between the cell and the surrounding medium.

Contrast can be enhanced either by staining, use of Dark Field or Phase Contrast Microscopy. In the process of   staining the specimen is treated with dyes that bind selectively either to the whole cell or certain cell components thus producing   a much greater absorption of incident light. Specific type of microorganisms and/or particular structures of microorganisms exhibit different staining reactions that can be readily distinguished. e.g. Gram stain or the acid fast stain is used to obtain information about the composition of cell wall layers of bacterial cells. In negative staining the stain e.g. India ink or   nigrosin 'does not enter the cell. This reveals the surface layers of very low refractive index such as capsules and slime layers surrounding microbial cells. (Fig. 1.8).

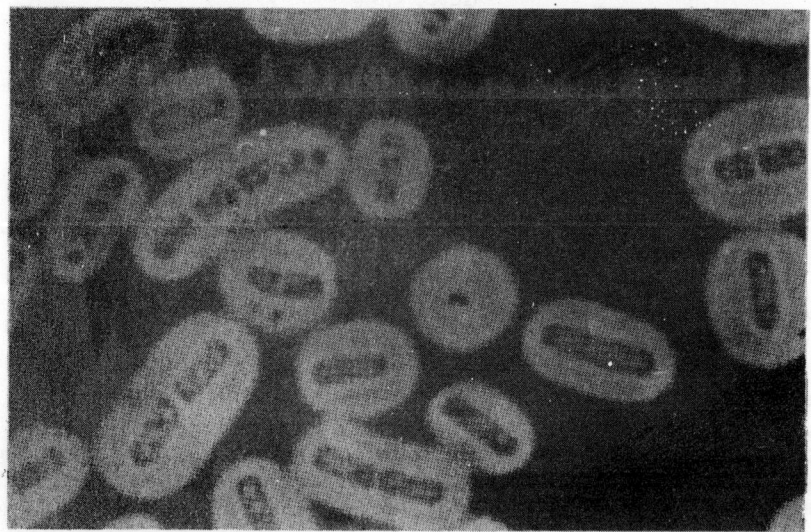

Fig. 1.8 : Bacterial capsules of *Bacillus meaterium* demonstrated by dispersing the cells in India in (x2, 160) Courtesy C.S. Robinow

2.3   Uses of the Light (Bright Field) Microscope

With a magnification of 1500 X   and a resolution of 100   -200 nm,the Light (Bright Field) microscope is a very useful tool for gross morphological observation of microorganisms ranging from 1-200 µm. This range includes bacteria, yeasts, molds, algae and protozoa among microorganisms and cells of tissues of several bacterial and zoological specimens.

Morphological examination of microorganisms can be put to a variety of uses. For example, the viewing of bacteria (except   cyanobacteria) requires special staining techniques which, not only help in visualising bacteria but also often forms the basis of their classification. As in the case of Gram staining which stains blue for Gram positive and pink for Gram negative cells. This gives information about the chemical nature of the cell wall and hence forms the basis of classification. It is also possible to see the characteristic sizes, shapes and arrangements that is if present as chains, clusters, or individual unicells (Fig. 1.9). Streptobacilli for example, appear as chains of rod-shaped cells while *E. coli* appear as rod-shaped individual cells .

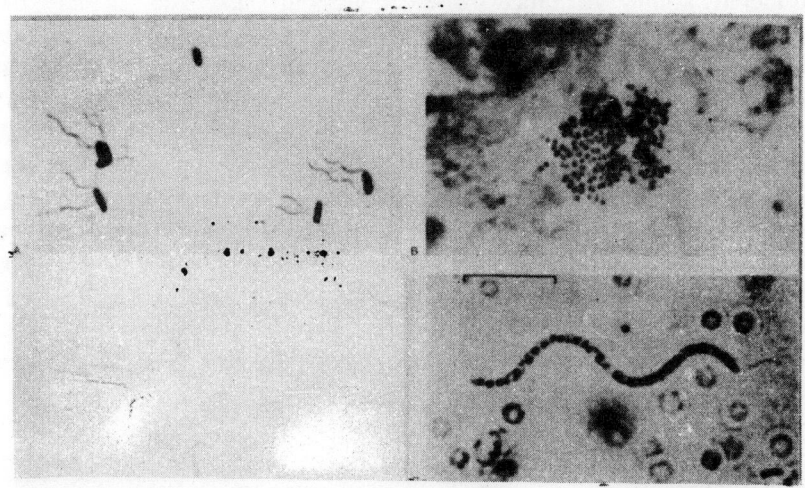

Fig. 1.9 : As revealed in these photomicrographs, by using bright field microscopy, the charecteristic sizes, shapes and arrangement of microbial cells can be obserrved (A) Rod shaped cells of *Bordella bronchiseptica* with flagella emanating from the cells (Courtesy Centre for disease Control Atlanta). [B] Cocal shaped cells of *Streptococcus viridans* (Courtesy John J. Bochino, Norton's Kosair Children's Hospital, Lousiville, Kentucky [c] Spiral shaped cells of *Thiovulum* sp. (Courtesy JWM la Riviere, International Institute for Hydraulic and Environmental Engineering Delft).

Occurence of fission, presence of endospores and other such features help to elaborate life cycles of bacteria. Purity of bacterial cultures is established by observation under the light microscope of a drop of bacterial suspension. Contamination is detected either as morphologically different bacteria or those that stain differently from what is expected out of the particular culture being examined. Using the hemocytometer to be explained later in the chapter, the number of bacteria in a sample can be estimated.

Again, with the ocularmeter and stage micrometer, the size of bacterium can be found out. Using the hanging drop technique the mode of motility of bacteria can be observed e.g. the vibratory movement of *Oscillatoria,* a cyanobacterium or the twisting movement of spirochaetes.

Using the nuclear stain, the chromatin material of a cell becomes visible. In a prokaryote this shows the location of the nucleus or its dividing condition during fission. In a eukaryote, the different stages of mitosis in a cell of a young dividing tissue can be seen.

Morphological observation of fungi, algae and protozoa, likewise, is used for classification, elaboration of lifecycles, modes of motility, finding the number and size of spores etc. As an example, the presence or absence of septa in a fungal mycelium separates the class Phycomycetes from higher fungi.

The anatomy of plant and animal tissue specimens is also studied principally under the light microscope. By simple observation of a blood smear on the slide, the heterogenous nature of the blood tissue can be understood. Treatment with antisera and subsequent observation under the microscope shows whether or not coagulation has occured thereby aiding the process of blood grouping.

The Light Microscope is thus, by far the most widely used microscope,due to its low cost, easy workability, and immense versatility. However due to its lower magnification and resolution as compared to the Electron Microscope (See Table 1.2), detailed examination of microorganisms or for that matter smaller microorganisms like myco-plasmas and viruses is not possible. Until the advent of the Electron Microscope, the great complexity of a eukaryotic cell was concealed since structures like the endoplasmic reticulum, golgi bodies, mitochondria, internal structure of chloroplasts cannot be seen through a Light Microscope. Also, since it has no system for enhancement of contrast it relies either on staining or on the intrinsic contrast of the specimen. Hence structures with low refractive index are difficult to stain e.g. slime sheaths around bacteria often go unnoticed. Under such circumstances one resorts to either Dark Field microscopy or Phase Contrast microscopy (Fig. 1.10).

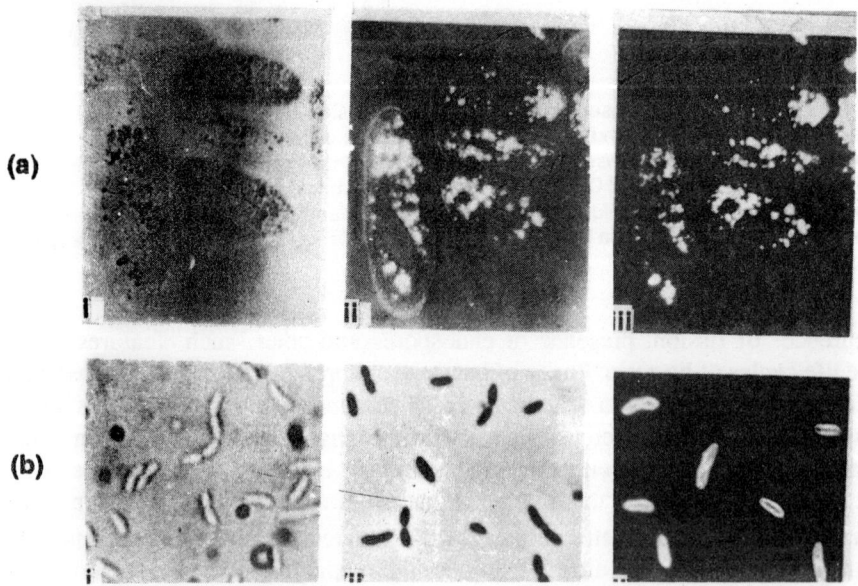

Fig. 1.10 (a) : Phase Contrast Microscopy compared with Bright Field and Dark Field Micros-copy. The same specimen of a protozoan seen by each method (i) Bright Field (ii) Phase COntrast (iii) Dark Field (Courtesy O.W. Richards, Research Deptt. American Optical Company).

Fig. 1.10 (b) : Photomicrographs of lining unstained Rod-shaped cells of *Pseudomonas fluorescens*. They can be seen indistinctly by Brright Field (i) but are readily visible by Phase Contrast (ii) or Dark Field Microscopy (iii) (Courtesy N.R. Kreig).

2.4 Care of the Microscope

If the Light Microscope has so much to offer us we, on our part, should take good care of it.

(i) The lens surface of eyepiece and objective should be wiped clean using either a lint free soft cloth or lens cleaning paper before and after use.

(ii) The lens covers should be duly replaced after use.

(iii) If however, fungal growth occurs on the lens, it should never be scratched with nails or a sharp instrument. It should be given to specialists who clean them by dipping them in special solutions.

(iv) The 100 X objective lens should never be used without oil.

(v) The microscope should be kept covered when not in use.

3. The Dark Field Microscope

The enhancement of contrast can be brought about not only by staining but also by using several alternative miroscope designs that do not require staining thereby permitting the visualisation of living specimens. The simplest of these microscopes is the Dark Field Microscope (Fig. 1.11). Many objects appear invisible against a bright background due to lack of contrast but are visible against a dark background. In order to obtain a dark back-ground, direct light which illuminates the objective must not enter the objective. This is accomplished by the use of a special condenser that transmits a hollow cone of light, apex down and through the specimen (Fig. 1.12). The diverging rays do not enter the objective. Only light scattered by the specimen enters the objective. Thus the specimen appears as a bright speck in a dark field. The special Dark Field condenser could be either the paraboloid or the cardiod type.It could also be the bright field condenser used with a dark field stop. (Fig. 1.13)

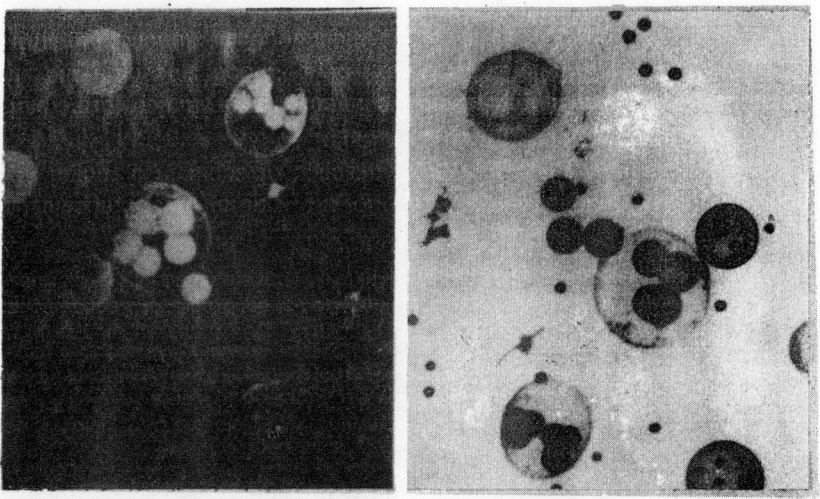

Fig. 1.11 : Dark Field Microscopy is useful for visualising microbial cells without the need for staining to enhance contrast. (a) Micrograph of a colony of green alga *Volvox* in dark field. Microscopy (b) Colony of *Volvox* in bright field microscopy.

(Courtesy Gary B. Collins, Usepa, Cincinnati).

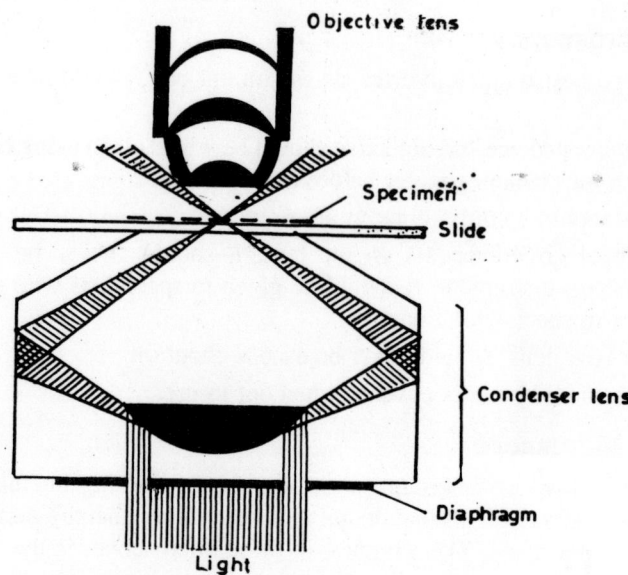

Fig. 1.12 : Schematic representation of dark field illumination.

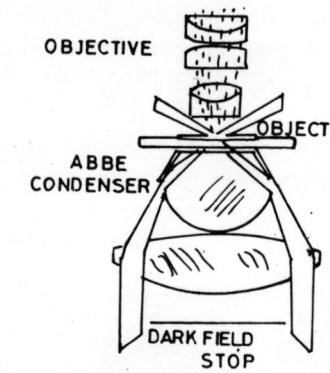

ABBE CONDENSER WITH DARKFIELD STOP

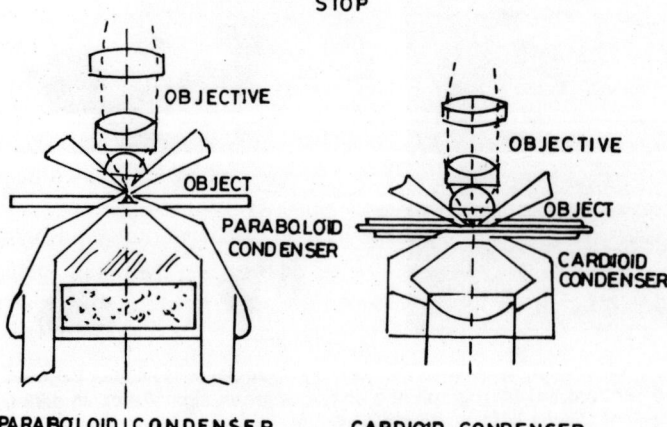

PARABOLOID CONDENSER   CARDIOID CONDENSER

Fig. 1.13 : Various forms of condensers for oblique illumination of the darkfield.

4. THE PHASE CONTRAST MICROSCOPE

Contrast between specimen and surrounding medium can also be increased by using a specialised microscope called the Phase Contrast microscope in which the optical system is modified. The phase contrast microscope optically converts differences in the speed with which light passes through a specimen into differences in contrast that can be seen. Like the Dark field microscope, it is useful for visualising living microorganisms and eliminates the necessity of staining to view microbial structures (Fig. 1.14).

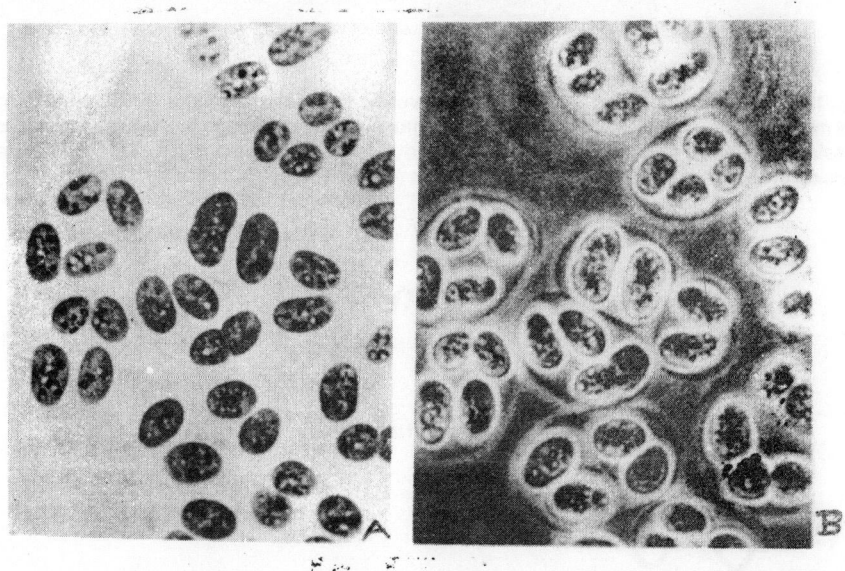

Fig. 1.14 : The cell structures in the photomicrograph from the phase contrast microscope **(a)** are easier to see as compared to the photomicrograph using brightfield **(b)** These are photomicrographs of the cyanobacterium *Gloecapsa* (From BPS-J. Robert Waaland Univ. of Washington).

This type of microscope relies upon the fact that light passing through a cell of higher refractive index (with a greater ability to change the direction of a ray of light) than the surrounding medium is slowed down relative to the light that passes directly through the less dense background medium. The greater the refractive index of the cell, the greater the retardation of the light wave (Fig. 1.15). Thus when light passes through a microorganism, there is a slight alteration in the phase of the light wave, i.e. the point of advancement within the light wave cycle. The conversion of differences in the phase of the light wave is based upon interference between light waves reaching the image plane. When two waves out of phase with each other by a phase difference of $\lambda/2$ reach the image plane they destructively interfere, cancel each other out and produce DARK-NESS. On the contrary two light waves in phase on reaching the image plane combine and reinforce each other to produce a wave of twice the amplitude, hence higher intensity, resulting in BRIGHTNESS (Fig. 1.16).

The Phase Contrast Microscope is designed to separate direct undiffracted background light from the light passing through the object and getting diffracted causing these two different waves to be approximately 90 out of phase with each other so that they destructively interfere at the image plane and cause changes in light intensity (Fig.

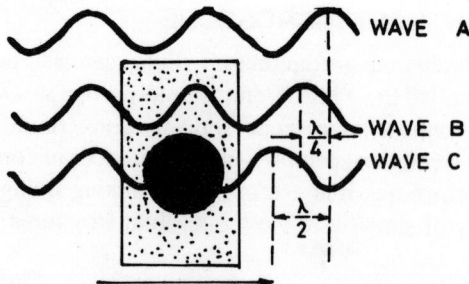

Fig. 1.15 : The Retardation of phases of light waves as they pass through a Transparent living cell mounted in saline. Compared to the waves that do not pass through the cell **(a)** The waves passing through the full thickness of the cytoplasm **(b)** Have been retarded by 1/4 *, and those passing through a more highly refractile inclusion **(c)** Have Been Retarded by 1/2 *

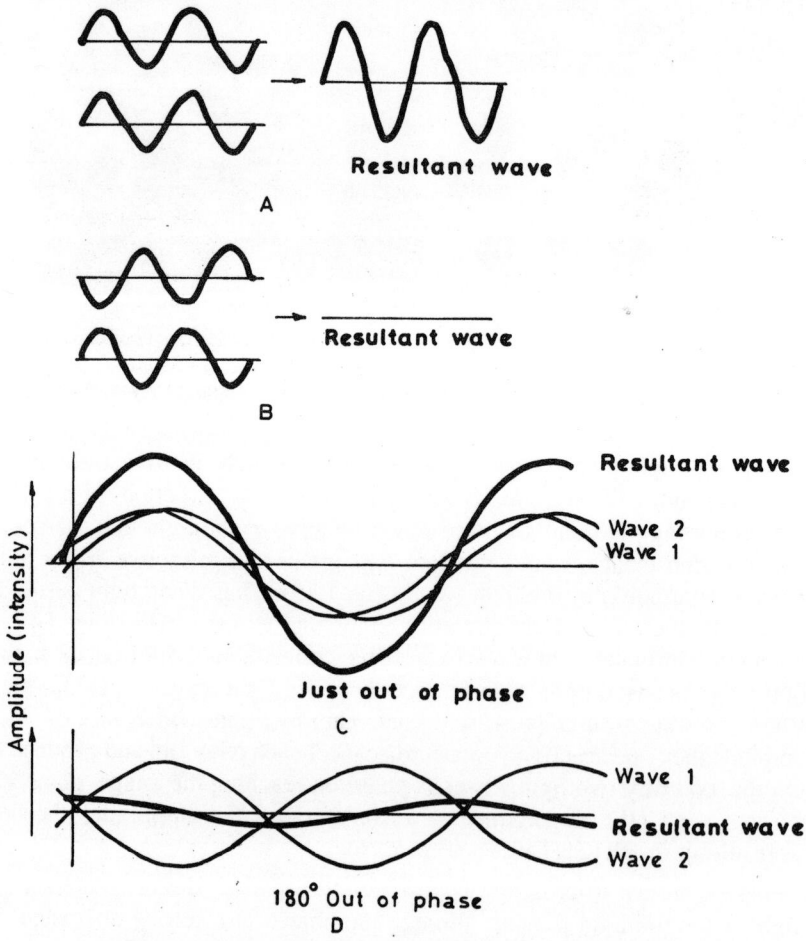

Fig. 1.16 : Additive and destructive interference of light waves.

1.17). **To** achieve this an annular diaphragm on the sub-stage condenser allows a ring of light to pass through the condenser and objective and fall on a corresponding ring-shaped area on a phase shifting plate placed on the back focal plane of the objective.

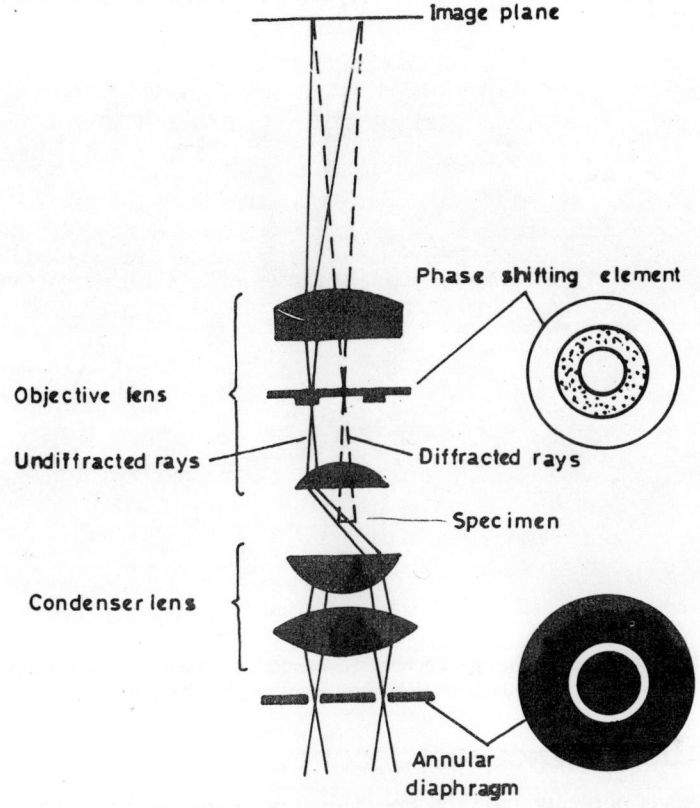

Fig. 1.17 : Schematic representation of the phase contrast microscope.

The ring-shaped area of the phase shifting plate is thinner than the rest of the plate so that rays passing through it are altered in phase by 90°, or $\lambda/4$. Rays which pass through the specimen directly, undiffracted, fall on this thin ring - shaped area and are advanced by 90° while those that are diffracted by the specimen pass through the thicker portion and are retarded by 90°. When these two waves recombine on the image plane ,they interfere destructively greatly increasing the contrast of the cells or intracellular structures that differ slightly in refractive index from their surroundings. The difference in phase increases contrast, hence a Phase Contrast Microscope.

5. INTERFERENCE MICROSCOPE

Like the Phase Contrast Microscope interference microscope is used for enhancing contrast. Both phase contrast and interference microscope utilise the fact that light travels as waves and that the addition of light waves that are out of phase with each other produces interference that alters the amplitude of light waves. While the Phase Contrast Microscope uses one beam of light that passes through the specimen, interference microscopes have two beams of plane polarised light that are combined after passing through the specimen These microscopes have higher Numerical Apertures, better contrast & can produce coloured pictures with vivid topographic relief. However because of their expense phase contrast microscope is the prefered method for observing wet mounts of bacteria. (Fig. 1.18).

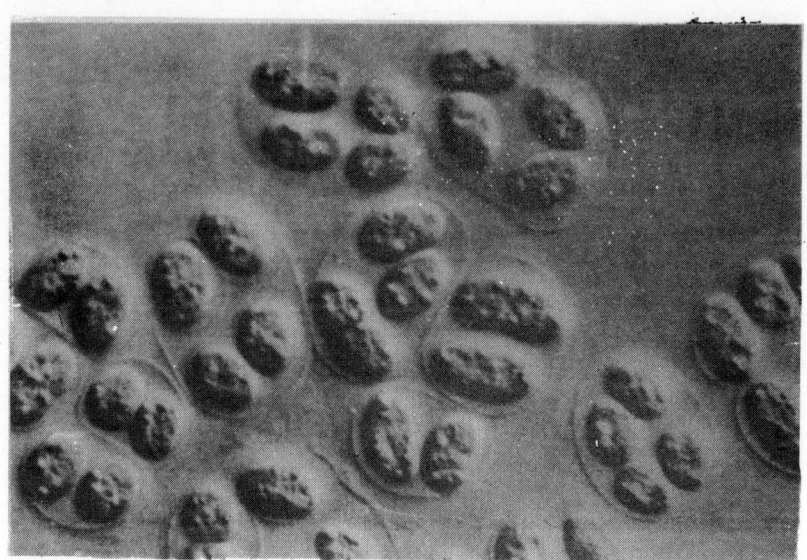

Fig. 1.18 : Photomicrograph of the cynobacterium *Gloeocapsa* using Nomarski Interference Microscopy (2, 800 x) (From BPS-J. Robert Waaland, Univ. of Washington).

6. UV AND FLUORESCENCE MICROSCOPE

The resolving power of the light microscope is directly related to the wavelength of light employed

$$d = 0.5 \ \lambda/N.A.$$

A slight improvement in resolution (about two fold) can be achieved by the use of an ultra-violet light source which has shorter wavelength than visible light. This is UV microscopy and the microscope is modified in that glass lenses are replaced by quartz lenses as glass is opaque to UV light. Also a camera is used to record the image since the eye cannot perceive UV light and in fact causes blindness. However, its complexity and expense have limited the use of UV microscopy. A modification called Fluorescence microscopy, having the same resolving power as UV microscopy, has come into limelight.

Microscopy that involves staining with fluorescent dyes is known as Fluorescence microscopy. When a fluorescent dye is illuminated by light of one wavelength-excitation wavelength, it gives off light of another wavelength-emission wavelength which is always shorter than excitation wavelength. The wavelength of light used to excite the dye maybe in UV range but the emitted light that is to be viewed must be in the visible range. The excitation light maybe transmitted either from below the specimen in which case it is called transmitted fluorescence, or to the specimen through the objective lens in which case the system is refered to as epifluorescence (Fig. 1.19) Fluorescence microscopes are equipped with various excitation filters that permit the selection of the wavelength used to illuminate the specimen and barrier filters that prevent all but the emission wavelength from reaching the ocular lens.

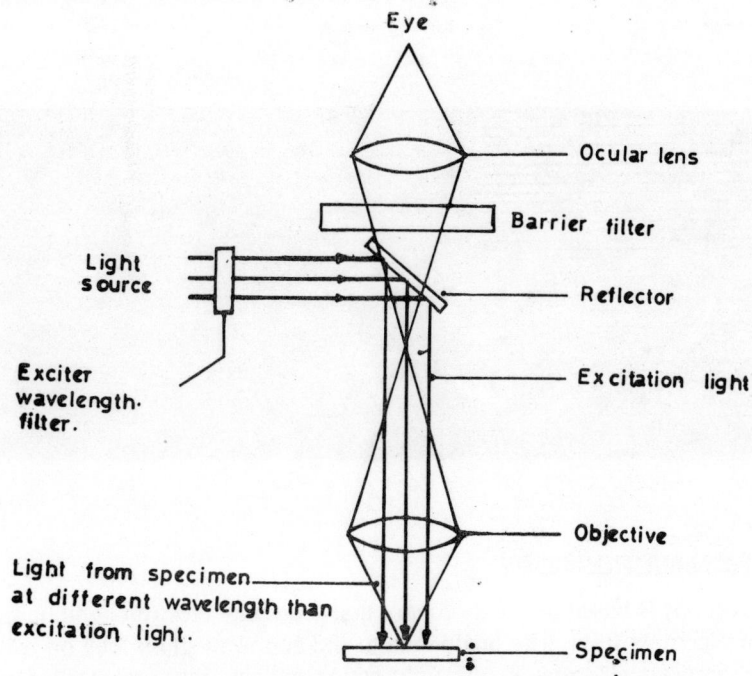

Fig. 1.19 : Diagram of an epifluorescence Microscope showing the light path.

6.1 Uses

An example of direct staining of bacteria with the fluorescent dye is shown in Fig1 1.20. The fluorescent dye auramine has astrong affinity for the wax-like substance of tubercle bacilli. The hard to find tubercle bacilli are stained with a uramine when they fluoresce with a brilliant yellow glow and diagnosis can be quickly made.

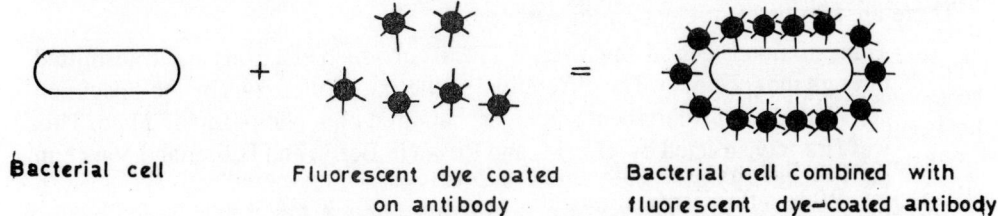

Bacterial cell   Fluorescent dye coated on antibody   Bacterial cell combined with fluorescent dye-coated antibody

Fig. 1.20 : Fluorescence staining technique and microscopy.

One of the reasons that Fluorescence Microscopy has become important in microbiology is that fluorescent dyes can be conjugated (linked) with antibodies (specific proteins produced against antigens as part of the immune response), providing great specificity in staining procedures. Antibodies to which a fluorescent dye is attached are referred to as labelled antibodies. These are mixed with a suspension of bacteria (antigen) and then the preparation can be examined by Fluorescent microscopy. The bacterial cells that have combined with the labelled antibody will be visible. This phenomenon is called immunofluorescence and is used immensely in diagnostic procedures (Fig. 1.21).

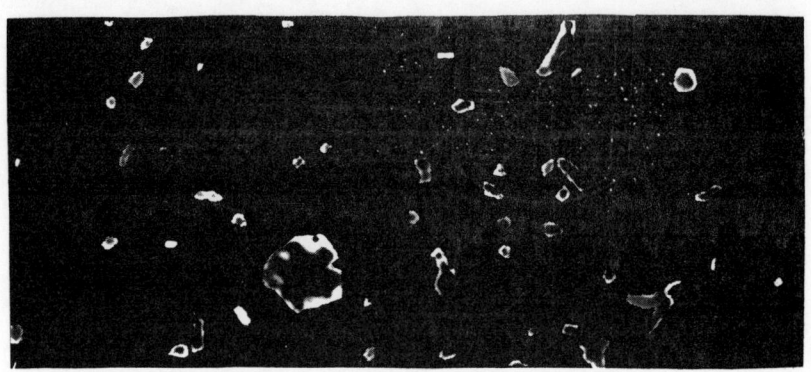

7. ELECTRON MICROSCOPY

Electron Microscopy is based on the discovery that a circular electromagmetic field acts on a beam of electrons in a way analogous to the action of glass lens on a beam of photons. The circular electromagnetic field acting as lens, is a lens coil formed by several thousand turns of wire in a soft iron casing. When current is made to pass through the coil a magnetic field is developed which directs movement of electrons. An electron beam has the properties of an electromagnetic wave of very short wavelength. When accelerated through an electric field, its wavelength (λ)

$$\lambda \alpha \quad 1 \, \sqrt{\text{accelerating voltage}}$$

With an accelerating voltage of 100 KV a wavelength of 0.04 nm (10,000 X shorter than visible light) is obtained. Consequently the resolving power increases and high useful magnification can be achieved.

There are two types of electron microscopy:

    (a) Transmission Electron Microscopy (TEM) in which electrons are transmitted through the specimen. The differential scattering of electrons by the specimen are viewed on a fluorescent screen or captured on a photographic plate. This was first constructed by Borries and Ruska in Berlin and Hillier and Vance in the U.S. in 1938.

    (b) Scanning Electorn Microscopy (SEM) in which the electrons are made to impinge on the specimen from above, the secondary electrons ejected are collected by a positively charged plate (anode) amplified and viewed on a cathode ray tube.

The number of secondary electrons ejected depends on surface topography of the specimen. Hence a three dimensional specimen is possible. This was first constructed in 1960 by Knoll et al.

7.1 Operation of the TEM

(A) Parts (Fig. 1.22)
   (i) Source/ electron gun
   (ii) Lens system and viewing
   (iii) Vacuum system
   (iv) Electronic system designed to hold electronic voltage stable.

(B) Sample prepartion
   (i) Fixing and dehydration
   (ii) Ultra Microtomy
   (iii) Staining
   (iv) Mounting

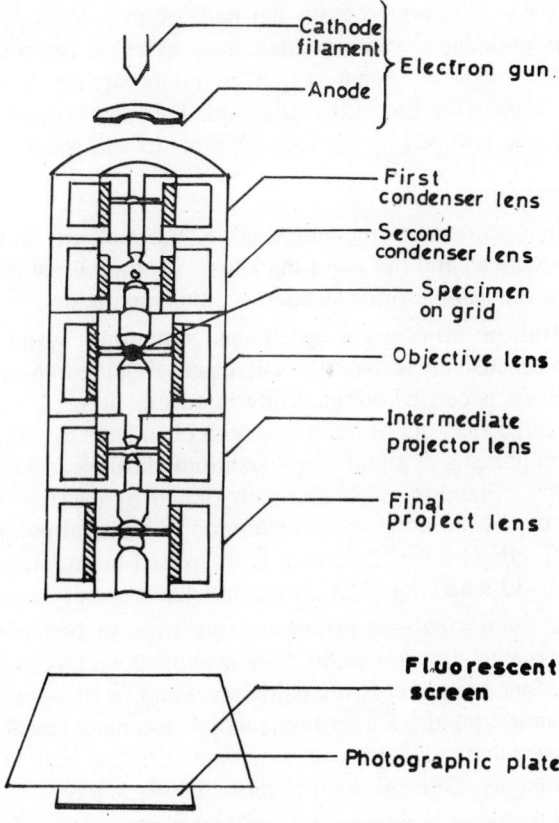

Fig. 1.22 : The tem allows the visualization of the fine detail of tthe microbial cell. **(a)** Diagram of a tem

(A) **Parts:**

Source : The source of electrons is a hot tungsten filament at 30 to 150 KV potential. Electrons are drawn from the filament and accelerated as a fine beam past an anode by a high voltage established between filament and anode.

Lens system and viewing : Analogous to the glass lens system   of the light microscope there is a magnetic lens coil system viz.

(a) Condenser lens coil system

(b) Objective lens coil system

(c) Intermediate projector

The condenser lens collimates the electron beam on the specimen by varying the current to the lens. After transmission through the specimen the objective lens coil focusses the electron beam   into a first (real) image of object enlarged about 2000X. The projector, like the eyepiece of the light microscope, magnifies a portion of the first image about 250,000 X total magnification and projects the image onto a fluorescent screen or film plate which is necessary because the electron beam cannot be viewed directly. The operator can look into the main tube by means of portholes or magnifying binocular glasses and can scan the images on the fluorescent screen, manipulate the objects and adjust alignment and field strength of the focussing magnets.

Vacuum system : Air is removed from the path of the electron beam to prevent collisions with gas molecules which scatter the electron beam and to reduce heat associated with the electron beam which would otherwise destroy the biological specimen and also reduce the life of the filament. This necessitates introduction of air locks for insertion and removal of photographic plates and specimens.

(B) Sample Preparation

The vacuum   system of the microscope, the lack of sufficient contrast in biological specimens and the extra thickness of microorganisms necessitates the preparation of the sample prior to microscopic examination.

Fixing and dehydration: Biological specimens containing water cannot be placed under high vacuum because the water will boil destroying the integrity of the specimen. Fixing and dehydration is carried out carefully in several stages (Fig. 1.23). Fixation is achieved either by rapid freezing or treatment with chemicals to stabilise and cross-link protein and lipid components of membranes. Osmium tetroxide is a common fixative for electron microscopy. Fixed tissue is then dehydrated by passing through increasing concentrations of ethanol. A more recent technique is 'critical point drying' in which, after treatment with ethanol, the specimen is immersed in pressurised liquid CO_2 and temperature raised to 32 when liquid CO_2 vaporises leaving a dry undistorted specimen.

Ultra Microtomy: Even microorganisms are too thick to be viewed under TEM therefore it is necessary to slice them into thin sections by a process called microtomy. In this process, the specimen after being dehydrated and fixed, is embedded in a plastic material for easy handling under a microtome which is a mechanical slicing instrument that moves a specimen across a knife with a diamond or glass edge. The plastic material is removed with solvents. The specimen is subsequently stained.

Staining: In TEM, contrast is produced by differential scattering of electrons by the specimen. Electron images are "shadows" produced mainly by the scattering of electrons. Scattering is produced when electrons encounter atoms. Heavy atoms like Au Pb^{207} U^{237} Os^{192} produce more scattering than light atoms C^{12}, N^{14} O^{16}. Since biological specimens are composed mainly of light atoms like C,N, O electron scattering and therefore contrast is very slight. Contrast can be greatly enhanced by "positive" staining that is combination of the organic matter in the cell with metals of high molecular weights Pb, U, Os, Au etc. Since they have   different weights and combine differently with different organic   compounds, their use permits a helpful degree of differential staining. In "negative" staining the background is stained with an   electron opaque material-material which scatters electrons-commonly phosphotungstic acid. This does not penetrate the cell but darkens the background.

Mounting: Instead of placing the specimen on a glass slide as is done in Light Microscopy, it is placed on a copper mesh grid within the evacuated column of the Electron Microscope. The specimen is sprayed onto a very thin film of electron transparent organic material like collodion which is then supported on the copper mesh grid.

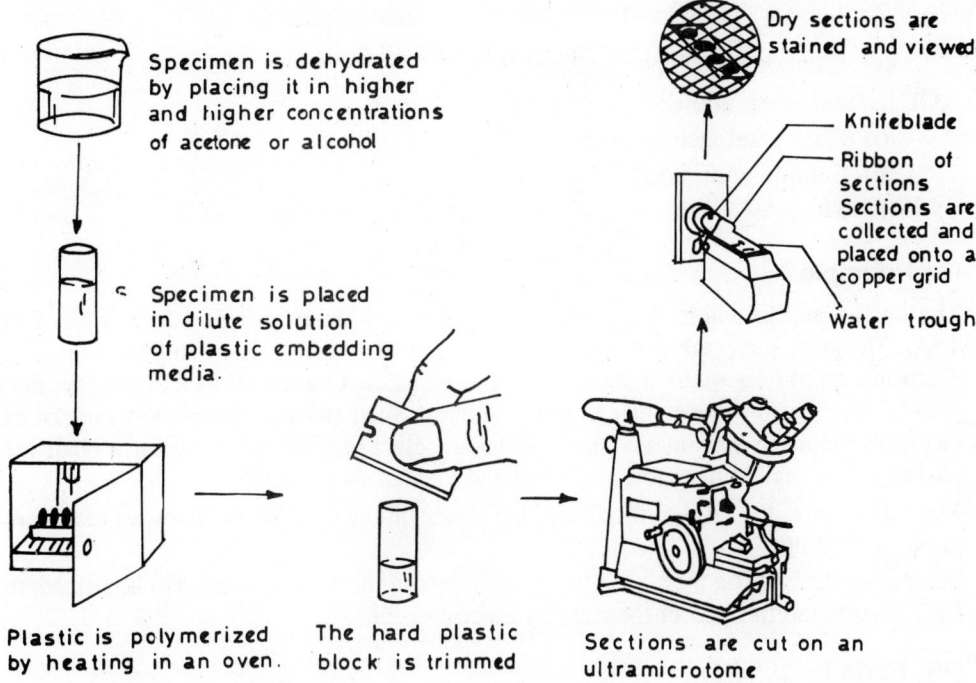

Specimen is dehydrated by placing it in higher and higher concentrations of acetone or alcohol

Specimen is placed in dilute solution of plastic embedding media.

Plastic is polymerized by heating in an oven.

The hard plastic block is trimmed

Sections are cut on an ultramicrotome

Dry sections are stained and viewed

Knifeblade

Ribbon of sections
Sections are collected and placed onto a copper grid

Water trough

Fig. 1.23 : Preparation of a specimen for viewing by Transmission Electron Microscopy.

7.1.1. Operational Problems.

Magnetic lenses suffer from problems similar to those found in glass lenses, though of electrical rather than of refractive origin, e.g. spherical and chromatic aberration caused by differences in electron velocities and energies.

A common problem is the appearance of artifacts which are not true representations of the specimen to be viewed. This is a problem common to all microscopes but particularly so in electron microscopes because of high magnifications that are used, improper dehydration of the specimen and improper adjustment of the electron beam.

7.1.2. Disadvantages

The most outstanding disadvantage for biological specimens is that they cannot be viewed live. The high energy electron beam falling on them and the necessary process of sample preparation kills the cell. With the sophistication required for such high magnification the cost of an electron microscope becomes prohibitively expensive.

7.2 Operation of the SEM

(A) Principle

(B) Parts

    (i) Source/Electron gun

    (ii) Condenser lens coil system

    (iii) Detector

    (iv) Amplifier

    (v) Cathode Ray Tube display (CRT)

(C) Sample Preparation

    (i) Fixing and Dehydration

    (ii) Coating with metal

    (iii) Mounting

(A) Principle

The operational principle and design of the SEM are quite different from that of the TEM. The principle combines the mechanism of electron microscopy and television. It is electronic amplification of signals generated by irradiating the surface of the specimen with a very narrow beam of electrons (probe). Such primary irradiation knocks off electrons from the specimen. These secondary electrons are collected on a positively charged plate called detector, amplified and viewed on a CRT.

Magnification is the ratio of the size of the image on the CRT to the diameter of the area scanned by probe.

Resolution depends on the size of the phosphorescent dots that are used to illuminate the CRT screen and the size of the primary electron beam.

(B) Parts (Fig. 1.24)

Source: An anode accelerates electrons generated or lanthanum hexabromide cathode at 30-150 KV potential.

Condenser lens coil system: The condenser lens coil system sharply focusses a fine beam of electrons on the specimen. Instead of forming an inverted cone of rays illuminating a wide field as in a light/TEM, electrons are made to form a needle sharp PROBE. The primary beam or probe acts as an exciter of image-forming secondary electrons that are ejected from the surface of the specimen. The number of electrons ejected depends on topography of the specimen. The probe scans the specimen in a raster pattern, like that on a blank TV screen.

Detector: The secondary electrons are magnetically deflected to a collector or detector which is a positively charged plate.

Amplifier: The successive signals from the detector are amplified and transmitted to a CRT. The CRT beam and scanning beam are synchronised so that the image on the CRT is an accurate reproduction of the scanning image.

The final image is really a series of pictures of different points on the specimen seen in such rapid succession as to provide for the eye, a unified view of the entire surface of the specimen.

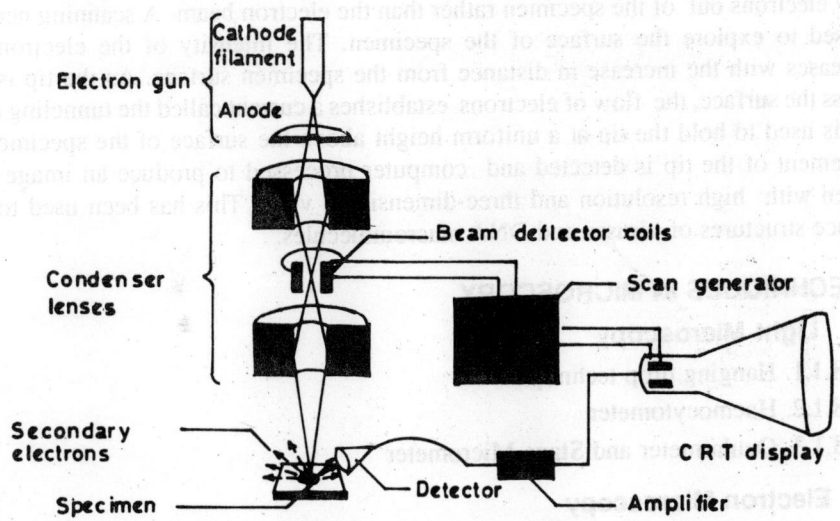

Fig. 124 : The sem is used for viewing surface structures and their three dimensional spatial Relationships.

(C) Sample Preparation

Fixing and Dehydration : As in the TEM, the electron fixing and dehydration beam in the SEM must be transmitted through a vacuum and therefore biological specimens must be fixed and dehydrated. The process being similar to that in TEM.

Coating with metal: Once the specimen is dehydrated it is covered by a thin film of metal like gold or gold palladium by vaporising the metal under vacuum and depositing it on the specimen. Coating with metal produces a conductive surface that permits dissipation of secondary electrons which otherwise create a surface charge on the non-conducting biological specimens. This distorts the image. After coating, specimens are mounted and viewed. Unlike TEM thin sectioning of specimen is unnecessary because only the surface structure of specimen is viewed.

7.2.1 Advantages and disadvantages of the SEM over the TEM

Since the intensity of secondary electron beam depends on the topography of the specimen, the CRT screen gives a three-dimensional appearance of the specimen. This is not possible in a TEM. However, the TEM has a better resolution (1nm) as compared to the SEM (10 nm), also, the TEM allows examination of internal structures of cells while the SEM does not, because the electron beam is not transmitted through the specimen. However, it is possible to expose and then view sub-surface layers by a technique called cryofracturing. In this, the specimen in frozen at very low temperatures, usually in liquid N_2 (-198°C) and then fractured with a sharp blade. The specimen fractures along planes that correspond to internal surfaces of the organism which can then be coated with metal and viewed.

7.3 Tunneling Electron Microscopy

The most recent technique in electron microscopy called Tunneling Electron Microscopy, won its inventors a Nobel prize in Physics in 1986. In this, magnets are used to draw electrons out of the specimen rather than the electron beam. A scanning needle tip is used to explore the surface of the specimen. The intensity of the electron cloud decreases with the increase in distance from the specimen surface. As the tip is swept across the surface, the flow of electrons establishes a current called the tunneling current that is used to hold the tip at a uniform height above the surface of the specimen. The movement of the tip is detected and computer processed to produce an image on the screen with high resolution and three-dimensional view. This has been used to view surface structures of viruses and DNA macromolecules.

8. TECHNIQUES IN MICROSCOPY

8.1   Light Microscopy

8.1.1. Hanging drop technique

8.1.2. Haemocytometer

8.1.3 Ocularmeter and Stage Micrometer

8.2 Electron Microscopy

8.2.1. Freeze etching and metal shadowing.

8.1.1 Hanging Drop Technique

Hanging drop technique enables viewing of size, shape, arrangement and motility of live microorganisms in fluid media. It requires the use of special ground slides (Fig. 1.25).

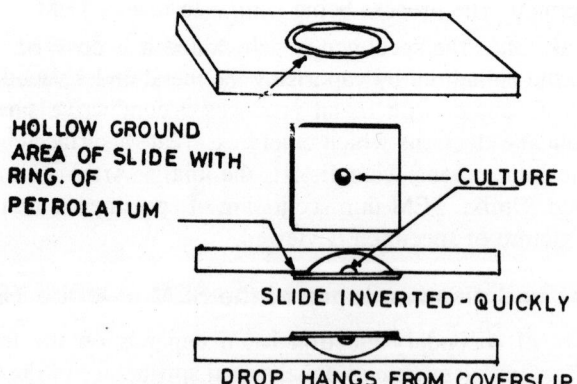

HOLLOW GROUND AREA OF SLIDE WITH RING. OF PETROLATUM

CULTURE

SLIDE INVERTED - QUICKLY

DROP HANGS FROM COVERSLIP

Fig. 125 : Hanging-drop-prepration.

In this technique, a loopful of bacterial suspension is placed in the centre of a cover slip. In the four corners tiny droplets of mineral oil are placed. The hollow ground slide is placed over the cover slip with the depression side down and the slide is inverted quickly so that the water cannot run off to one side. However, the lack of contrast yields limited though valuable information.

8.1.2 Haemocytometer

The haemocytometer, devised originally for counting haemocytes can be used for counting the number of bacteria, fungal spores etc. in a given volume of sample. The haemocytometer is a glass slide with a central area partitioned off by ridges into regular cubicle chambers of exactly known volume (Fig. 1.26). By counting the individual cells in each chamber under a microscope and adding them up, the number of organisms, living and dead may be computed.

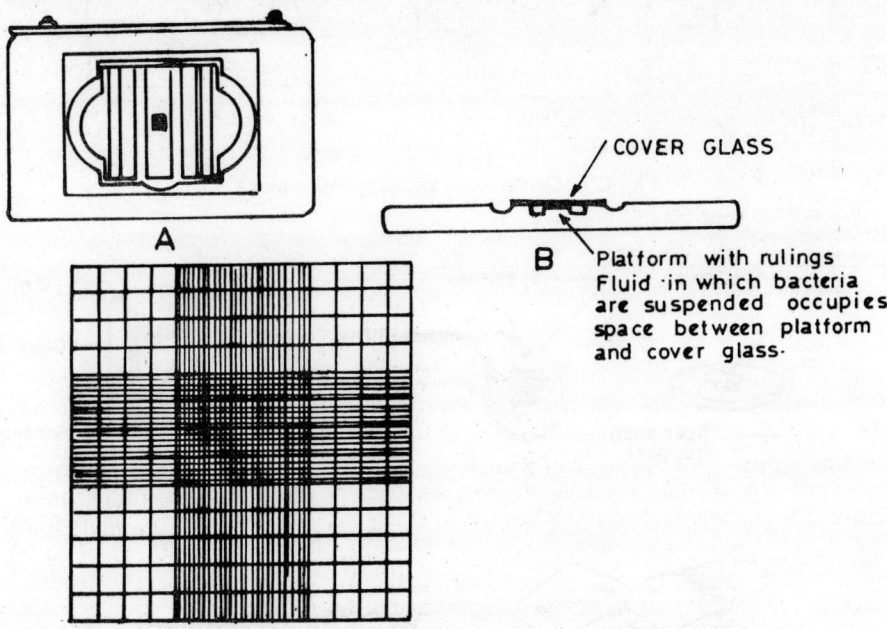

COVER GLASS

A

B

Platform with rulings
Fluid in which bacteria
are suspended occupies
space between platform
and cover glass.

Fig. 1.26 : A hemocytometer adapted for counting bacteria and other microgranisms. **(a)** Plan view showing dark central square covered by ruled chambers which are seen enlarged in c. **(b)** vertical section with cover glass in place.

8.1.3. Ocularmeter and Stage Micrometer for Micrometry

This is a technique in which the microscope is calibrated so that the size of objects being viewed can be found out. It involves the use of an ocularmeter or eye piece micrometer and a stage micrometer or object micrometer (Fig. 1.27).

The following operations are performed in sequence:

1. The eye piece is removed from the microscope and ocularmeter inserted between the lens and the diaphragm.
2. The stage micrometer is viewed through this eye piece
3. The number of divisions of the eyepiece and stage micrometer is noted.

   Say, x divisions of stage micrometer = y divisions of ocularmeter x/y divisions of stage micrometer = 1 division of ocularmeter. x/y is called the least count.
4. The stage micrometer is then replaced by slide with specimen.

5. The number of divisions of the ocularmeter which are equal to length of object to be measured is observed.

6. This value is then multiplied the least count to give the size of the object.

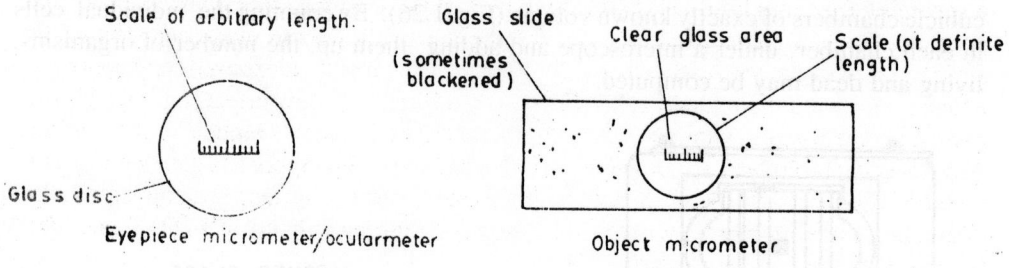

Fig. 127 : Ocularmeter and stage micrometer

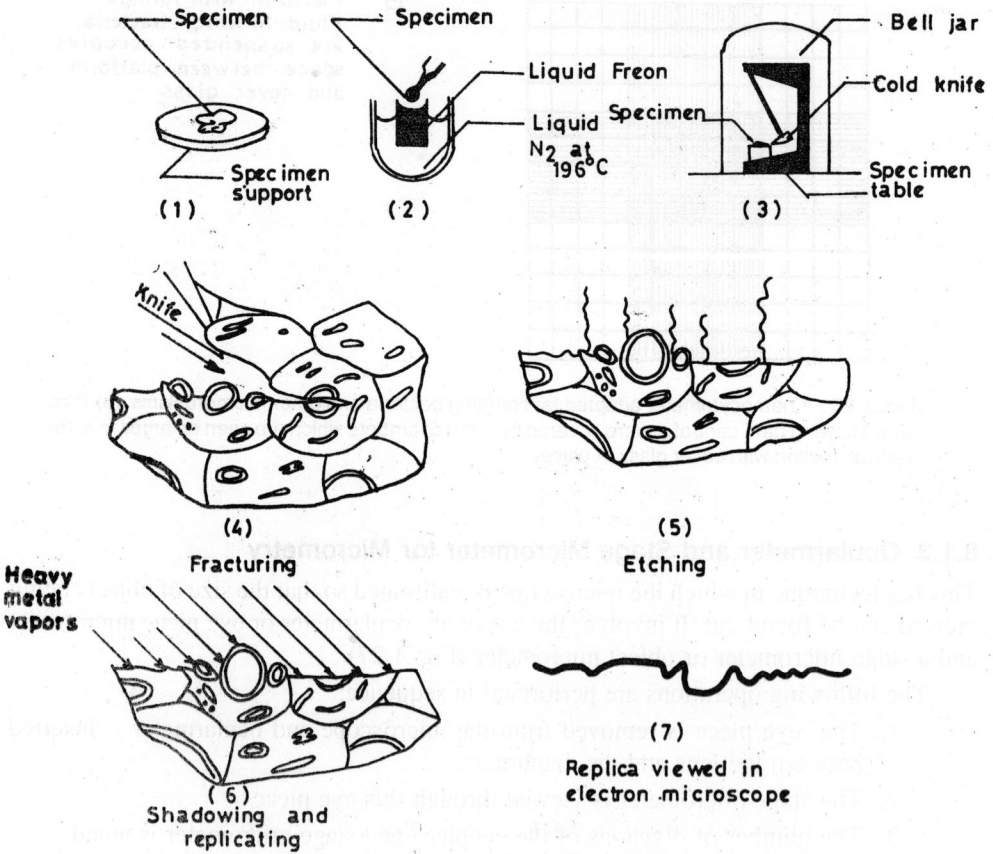

Fig. 1.28 : Procedure for the formation of Freeze-Fracture replicas used for visualising surface structure in conjunction with transmission electron microscopy.

8.2 ELECTRON MICROSCOPY

8.2.1. Freeze etching and metal shadowing

Freeze etching is used to reveal detailed structures of microorganisms. In this procedure a specimen frozen in liquid N_2 is fractured by striking it with a knife blade; the fractured specimen is then etched, that is, some of the ice is allowed to evaporate, raising the surface layer of the specimen (Fig. 1.28). The specimen is then exposed to vapours of a heavy metal while being held at 45° angle to produce a shadow effect, after which it is rotated and exposed to vaporised carbon at 90° angle to produce a replica of the surface. Any adhering biological specimen is removed and the carbon replica is then viewed.This method reveals much detail of both internal and external surface structures and also eliminates some problems with artifacts that arise through chemical fixation and sectioning of biological specimen.

2

CHROMATOGRAPHY

1. INTRODUCTION

What may be called chromatographic effects were being put to use some two thousand years ago. Dyers were accustomed to judge the quality of their dyes, and in particular to detect the presence of adulterants by letting a drop of solution spread out on a piece of cloth or paper (Papyrus). The fringe of colours formed at the boundary of the spot was usefully diagnostic. This, could be the roots of paper chromatography. Around the same time, column chromatography also took birth in the oil industry where crude oils were purified by allowing them to percolate through beds of carbon. However, as with many great discoveries the exact originator of the process could not be pointed out, though a few can be appreciated for giving due importance to the process by using it for separation, purification and identification of compounds. The first to give convincing evidence of the power and versatility of the process was M.S. Tswett, a botanist, who in 1906, isolated the principle plant pigments by passing them, in solution in petroleum ether through a column of powdered chalk. Chromatography based on differential partition between two immiscible solvents was first described, in 1941, by A.J.P. Martin and R.L.M. Synge. In this water was fixed within silica gel, mobile phase was chloroform and amino acids of a protein were analysed. Subsequently other classes of compounds e.g. antibiotics were analysed. Today, the technique has developed in all dimensions as perhaps the most powerful single analytical and preparative method available in the laboratory.

2. GENERAL PRINCIPLES

The basis of all forms of chromatography is differential partition of a compound between two immiscible phases, one of which is stationary and the other, mobile. The way in which a compound is partitioned or distributed between the two immiscible phases is given by the Partition Coefficient (K_d)

$$K_d = \frac{\text{Concentration in phase A}}{\text{Concentration in phase B}}$$

The value of K_d is constant at a given temperature.

Depending on the different types of phases involved there are following forms of chromatography (Table 2.1).

Table 2.1

Form phase	Mobile phase	Stationary phase	Principle of separation
1. Adsorption or Solid- liquid Chromatography	Liquid	Solid	Adsorption equilibrium between stationary solid and mobile liquid phases
2. Liquid-liquid or Partition Chromatography	Liquid	Liquid	Partition equilibrium between a stationary liquid & mobile liquid phase
3. Gas- liquid Chromatography	Gas	Liquid	Partition equilibrium between a stationary liquid & mobile gaseous phase.
4. Ion exchange Chromatography	Elect- rolyte	Ion ex- change	Ion exchange equilibrium between ion exchangeres inresin stationary phase & mobile electrolyte phase
5. Exclusion Chroma- tography/Gel filtration or Permeation Chro- matography	Liquid	Liquid	Molecular sieve action of pores of gel particles
6. Affinity Chromatography	Liquid containing macromole-	Ligand	Biological specificity & reversibility of binding between macromolecules and ligand.

Table 2.1 Depending on the mode by which separation is achieved there are three types of chromatography.

(1) Column Chromatography in which the stationary phase is packed   into glass or metal columns and the mobile phase percolates   through the column.

(2) Paper Chromatography in which the stationary phase is supported by cellulose fibres of paper and mobile phase moves   through the interstitial spaces by capillary action. Sometimes, the cellulose fibres of paper themselves act as solid stationary phase.

(3) Thin Layer Chromatography in which the stationary phase is thinly coated onto glass plates and mobile phase moves along it.

3. COLUMN CHROMATOGRAPHY

In the column technique the components of a mixture are separated in the column as distinct zones and each zone is eventually displaced from the column as a series of fractions (Fig. 2.1).

The apparatus and general techniques used for Column Adsorption, Partition, Ion exchange, Exclusion and Affinity Chromatography have much in common and are discussed below. GLC & HPLC have their own unique apparatus and procedures and are discussed separately.

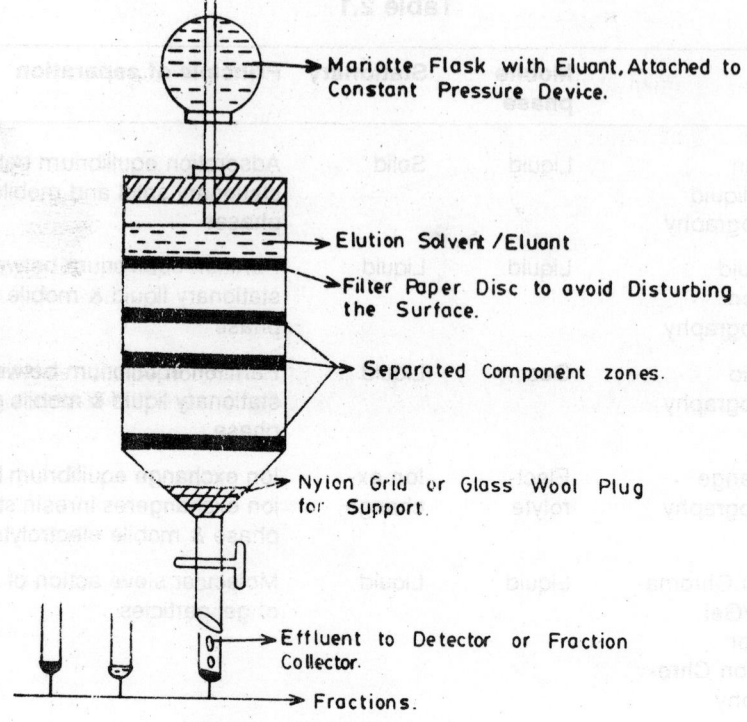

Mariotte Flask with Eluant, Attached to Constant Pressure Device.

Elution Solvent / Eluant

Filter Paper Disc to avoid Disturbing the Surface.

Separated Component zones.

Nylon Grid or Glass Wool Plug for Support.

Effluent to Detector or Fraction Collector.

Fractions.

Fig. 2.1 : Column Chromatography

3.1 Columns

Chromatography columns are usually glass and generally long columns give good resolution of components but wide columns are better for separation of large quantity of material. The essential features of a chromatography column are shown in Fig. 2.1. The glass column should have a means of supporting the stationary phase as near to the base of the column as possible to minimise the dead space below the column support in which post column mixing of separated compounds could occur. Commercial columns possess either a porous glass plate fused onto the base of the column or a suitable device for supporting a replaceable nylon net which in turn supports the stationary phase over it. Often glass wool plugs are used.

3.2 STATIONARY PHASES

Depending on the particular form of chromatography to be carried out there are different types of stationary phases e.g. solids (alumina, silica etc.) for adsorption chromatography, liquids for Partition Chromatography, gels for Exclusion Chromatography and resins for Ion-exchange Chromatography. All materials need to be equilibrated with the mobile liquid phase called solvent, before preparing the column. During equilibration the solid support material is allowed to settle and fine particles remaining in suspension are removed by decantation (Fig. 2.2a).

If this is not carried out the flow rate of the mobile phase will be considerably reduced due to clogging by these fine particles. In addition, some form of pretreatment of stationary phase is often required e.g. some gel filtration materials need to be swollen, adsorbents need to be activated by heating or acid treatment and ion-exchange resins have to be obtained in the required ionised form by washing.

3.3 Packing of columns

The chromatography column is packed with stationary phase (adsorbent , resin or gel) by pouring a slurry of the stationary phase in the mobile phase, into the column over a glass rod (Fig. 2.2b). This prevents trapping of air bubbles. Gentle tapping or stirring in the upper part of the slurry also ensures that no air bubbles are trapped and helps in even packing. Poor column packing gives rise to uneven flow (channeling) and reduced resolution. The slurry is added until the required height is obtained. The suspension is then allowed to settle and excess mobile phase is allowed to run off by opening the outlet. The column is then washed with the mobile phase and level of the liquid is kept just above the surface of the material. To prevent the column from being disturbed either by addition of

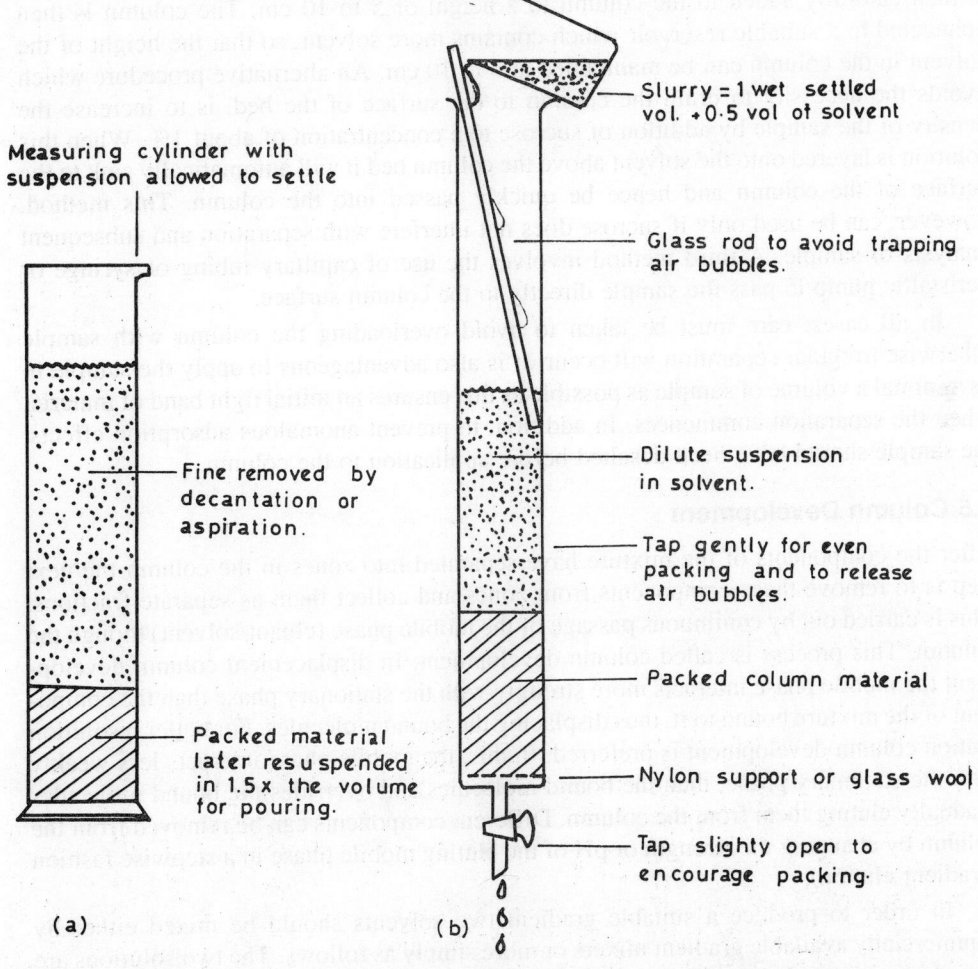

Measuring cylinder with suspension allowed to settle

Fine removed by decantation or aspiration.

Packed material later resuspended in 1.5 x the volume for pouring.

(a)

Slurry = 1 wet settled vol. + 0.5 vol of solvent

Glass rod to avoid trapping air bubbles.

Dilute suspension in solvent.

Tap gently for even packing and to release air bubbles.

Packed column material

Nylon support or glass wool

Tap slighty open to encourage packing.

(b)

Fig. 2.2 : The preparation of a chromatography column.

the mobile phase or during application of sample to the column, a filter paper disc or nylon or rayon gauze is placed on the surface of the column. Some commercial columns have an adaptor or plunger which serves the dual purpose of protecting the surface and providing an inlet (often capillary tubing) to carry the solvent to the column surface. Once a column has been prepared no part of it should be allowed to run dry i.e., a layer of mobile liquid should always be maintained above the column surface.

The total volume of the solid and liquid in the column is referred to as the bed volume and the volume of liquid phase outside the solid is called Void Volume (Vo).

3.4 Application of Sample

Several methods are available for the application of the sample to the top of the prepared column. A simple way is to remove most of the solvent from above by suction and just to drain the remainder into the column bed.The sample is then carefully applied by pipette and it too allowed just to run into the column. A small volume of solvent is then applied in a similar manner to wash final traces of the sample into the bed. More solvent is then carefully added to the column to a height of 5 to 10 cm. The column is then connected to a suitable reservoir which contains more solvent, so that the height of the solvent in the column can be maintained at 5 to 10 cm. An alternative procedure which avoids the necessity to drain the column to the surface of the bed, is to increase the density of the sample by addition of sucrose to a concentration of about 1%. When this solution is layered onto the solvent above the column bed it will automatically sink to the surface of the column and hence be quickly passed into the column. This method, however, can be used only if sucrose does not interfere with separation and subsequent analysis of sample. A third method involves the use of capillary tubing or syringe or peristaltic pump to pass the sample directly to the column surface.

In all cases, care must be taken to avoid overloading the column with sample otherwise irregular separation will occur. It is also advantageous to apply the sample in as minimal a volume of sample as possible as this ensures an initial tight band of material when the separation commences. In addition, to prevent anomalous adsorption effects, the sample should have been desalted before application to the column.

3.5 Column Development

After the components of the mixture have separated into zones in the column the next step is to remove these components from zones and collect them as separate fractions. This is carried out by continuous passage of the mobile phase (eluant/solvent) though the column. This process is called column development. In displacement column development the mobile phase interacts more strongly with the stationary phase than the component of the mixture bound to it, thus displacing the bound molecules. For better resolution elution column development is preferred. In this, the mobile phase interacts less weakly with the stationary phase, than the bound molecules and overrides the bound molecules gradually eluting them from the column. Different components can be removed from the column by changing the strength or pH of the eluting mobile phase in a stepwise fashion (gradient elution).

In order to produce a suitable gradient two solvents should be mixed either by commercially available gradient mixers or more simply as follows. The two solutions are placed in separate chambers. The recipient chamber is linked to the column and the donor chamber is linked to the recipient chamber by a siphon. As the eluant enters the column from the recipient chamber, the solution in the donor replaces it and is mixed by a stirrer. The diameter of the two chambers determines whether the gradient varies with time in a linear, convex or concave manner. Gradient elution, achieves better resolution as compared to isocratic elution which uses a single solvent as eluant. The volume of eluant required to elute a particular solute is known as elution volume (Ve) whilst the corresponding time for elution is known as the retention time (tr).

During elution it is essential that the flow rate should be maintained constant. This is achieved by gravity feed most simply. The flow rate may be regulated by adjusting the operating pressure which corresponds to the difference between the level of the solvent in a reservoir situated above the column and the level at the outlet side of the column. An ordinary open reservoir is not satisfactory as the operating pressure will drop as the solvent level drops while it runs through the column. A Mariotte flask (Fig. 2.1) can keep the pressure constant. Alternatively a peristaltic pump can pump the eluant at a predetermined rate onto the column. Care may be taken to see that the column structure does not change due to excessive pressure from the pump.

3.6 Fraction Collection and Analysis

As the components of a mixture emerge from the column as the effluent it is necessary to detect their presence in order to enable them to be isolated for further study. This can be done in two ways. In one, the effluent can be continiously monitored and in the other it can be collected as separate fractions which are subsequently analysed.

In continuous monitoring, the effluent is passed through a flow cell (8 mm^3) located in the detector. Detection may be based on UV or visible absorption by components at characteristic wavelengths, fluorescence, changes in the refractive index of effluent, the presence of a radioactive label, or the ease of oxidation or reduction as measured by an electrochemical detector. The signal generated by the detector is recorded on a chart recorder each emerging compound giving a characteristic peak from which it is possible to calculate the retention time and/or the elution volume (Fig. 2.3).

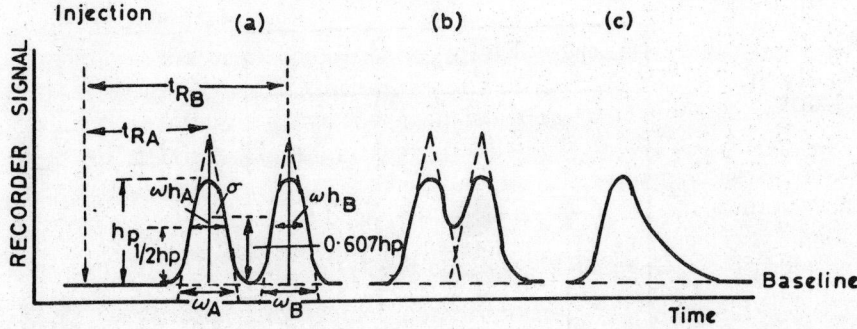

Fig. 2.3 (a) : Chromatogram of two compounds showing complete resolution and the calculation of retention times (b) Two compounds giving incomplete resolution and the production of fused peaks; (c) A compound showing excessive tailing.

Separate fractions can be collected either manually or by automatic fraction collection. The amount of effluent in each fraction can be determined in one of the several ways. There may be a siphoning system to deliver a predetermined volume into each tube or there may be an electronic means of allowing a predetermined number of drops to enter each tube. This has the disadvantage that if the composition of the effluent changes during gradient elution, its surface tension and therefore the size of drops may also change, so that the volume of liquid collected changes. In another method, the effluent is allowed to enter a tube for a fixed interval of time. But if the flow rate of column varies, the volume of fraction collected also varies. However, once the fractions have been collected they can be detected by spectrophometry, fluorimetry, scintillation counting and radioimmunoassay.

Quantitative estimations of the fractions collected can also be made using the peak area. The area of the peak is the product of the height of the peak (hp) and its width at half height (w_{hA}). The peak area can be shown to be proportional to the amount of sample component present. Alternatively, the peak may be cut out, weighed and the assumption made that area and weight are linearly related. The amount of the specific component can be found by a standard curve made by chromatographing the known sample under identical conditions and weighing the peak cut-out.

4. PAPER CHROMATOGRAPHY (PC) AND THIN LAYER CHROMATOGRAPHY (TLC)

4.1 Principle

Unlike Column Chromatography the components of the mixture after separation remain on the chromatogram in PC and TLC. On spraying with the appropriate detecting agent they appear as a series of spots. The position of spots is recorded in terms of the R_f value (Fig. 2.4). This is defined as the ratio.

$$R = \frac{\text{Distance moved by component}}{\text{Distance moved by mobile liquid phase/solvent.}}$$

R_f values are constant for a particular component under particular conditions.

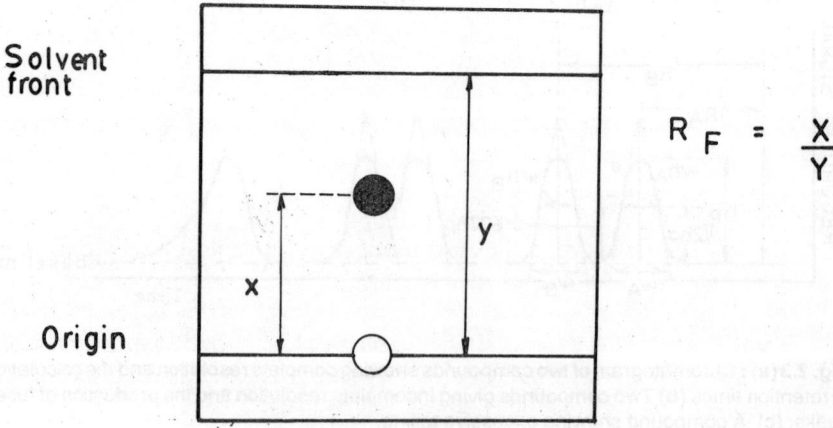

Fig. 2.4 : Finding the R_F Valve

In PC the stationary phase is supported by cellulose fibres of paper and the mobile phase moves through the interstitial spaces by capillary action. If paper merely acted as an inert support separation of components of a mixture would be exclusively due to continuous partition between mobile phase flowing along the paper and water held in the paper; filter paper contains 15% of its weight of water and this may be the case in some circumstances. More usually the paper affects separation in a number of ways; it acts as adsorbent especially for polar molecules for which it has great affinity. They are held by hydrogen bonding and Van der Waal's forces it functions also as an Ion-exchange material due to its content of carboxyl groups.

In TLC, a slurry of the stationary phase, generally in water, is applied to a glass, plastic or foil plate as a uniform thin layer by a plate spreader starting from one end and moving to the other. A variety of materials can be used as stationary phase and like PC, separation is achieved by multifarious ways. On heat activated layers of silica gel and similar substances, when non-aqueous solvent systems are used adsorption is the predominant process and this has been useful for separating hydrophobic substances such as lipids. When aqueous solvents are used on layers of crystalline material of large surface area and fine particle size, a situation between these two extremes exists and the magnitude of the influence of the inndividual components is difficult to assess.

4.2 Paper

Whatman number 1 is the paper most frequently used for analytical purposes. Whatman No. 3 MM is thick paper and is best employed for separating large quantities of material. The resolution is however, inferior to that of Whatman No. 1. For a rapid separation Whatman No. 4 & 5 are convenient though spots are less well defined. In all cases, the flow rate is faster in the machine direction which is normally noted on the box containing the papers. The paper may be impregnated with materials like silica for adsorption another liquid for partition chromatography etc. Silica impregnated papers are available commercially and are used for separation of lipids and hydrophobic molecules.

4.3 Thin Layer Preparation

A slurry of the stationary phase in water is applied evenly onto the plate. Often calcium sulphate is incorporated into the slurry to facilitate adhesion of the thin layer on the plate. For analytical purposes a layer of 0.25 mm thick is desired. For preparative separations 5 mm thick plates are used. With the exception of Thin Layer Exclusion Chromatography the plates are dried to leave a coating of the stationary phase. In the case of adsorbents, drying is carried out in an oven at 100 C - 120 C. This also serves to activate the adsorbent.

4.4 Sample Application

A drop of the solution containing the mixture of compounds to be separated is placed near one end of the strip by means of a syringe, capillary or micropipette. It is then allowed to dry at room temperature. The strip is then placed so that the end with the spot dips into the solvent which is the mobile liquid phase and moves by capillary action. The mobile liquid phase is usually a mixture of solvents. It is essential that the spot is not immersed in the solvent as it would dissolve and be lost.

4.5 Development

It is essential to make sure that prior to development the atmosphere of the separation chamber is fully saturated with the solvent, otherwise R values will vary from chamber to chamber. The process is called equilibration and is carried out as follows. About 1.5cm of mobile phase/solvent is added to the chamber and covered with a lid for at least half an hour. Unless this is done, irregular running of solvent will occur as it ascends the plate resulting in poor separations. After equilibration the lid is removed and the strip is placed inside, the spot slightly over the solvent. Whenever the solvent reaches the far end of the strip, or after a convenient time period the sheet is removed, rapidly dried and spots are detected by spraying a suitable locating agent on it. When a mixture contains many components, complete separations on a strip of finite length may not be possible. In order to overcome this difficulty a number of different solvents with different properties are used so that components running together in one solvent will probably separate in another solvent. Although many one-way chromatograms, each in a different solvent could be compared, a great deal more information is obtained if two solvents are used in conjunction to prepare a two-way chromatogram than if the two are used to prepare two one-way separations (Fig. 2.5).A two-way chromatogram is prepared by placing a drop of the mixture near a corner of a square or rectangular sheet of paper or layer. Solvent is then allowed to travel up with the result that a one way separation is obtained. After drying completely, the sheet is turned at right angles and run in a second solvent which performs a furthe separation and causes the components to be distributed on the sheet in two dimensions instead of the previous one dimension. This technique is called two - dimensional chromatography.

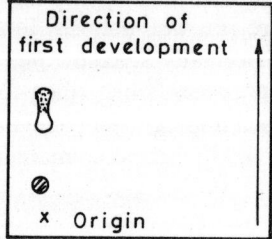 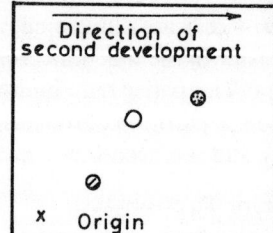

Fig. 2.5 : A two-dimensional chromatogram

There are two techniques which can be employed for the development of paper chromatograms - ascending and descending (Fig. 2.6). In both cases the solvent is placed at the base of a sealed tank or glass jar to allow the chamber to become saturated with solvent vapour. In the ascending method, the end of paper with the spot is dipped in the solvent at the base of the tank and as the solvent rises up — ascends — by capillary action, separation is achieved. In the descending technique the end of the paper with the spot is held in a through at the top of the tank and the rest of the paper allowed to hang vertically but not in contact with the solvent at the base of the tank. The solvent moves down from the trough — descends — under the force of gravity and separation is achieved. Though this achieves faster flow rates, it is not preferred because it is far more cumbersome to set up than ascending technique.

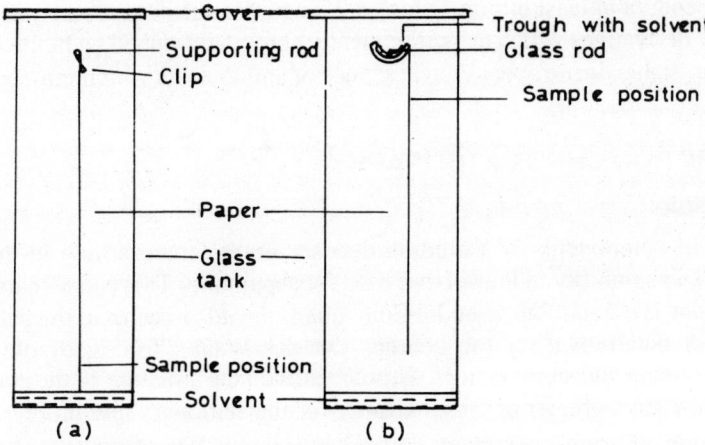

Fig. 2.6 : Ascending and (b) Descending methods of paper chromatography.

4.6 Component detection

Relatively few compounds are naturally coloured, fluoresce or absorb ultraviolet light and so after separation, majority of compounds are detected with a chemical location reagent.

The term 'location reagent' is defined as the total material applied to the dry chromatogram, after chromatography, in order to locate or reveal the positions of the separated substances so that a colour is produced which is different to that produced when the reagent is applied to a blank sheet which has also been run in the solvent. Thus the reagent includes: the chemicals (active constituents) which react to produce the colour, the solvent in which they are dissolved and any subsidiary substance which is added to strengthen or stabilise the colours so produced. Chemical reagents of this type suffer from the disadvantage, when compared to physical location methods (fluorescence, radioactivity, UV light, etc.) that they destroy the compounds being located.

4.7 Advantages of TLC over PC

A variety of supporting media could be used in TLC so that separation could be achieved in a variety of ways; adsorption, partition, exclusion, ion -exchange depending on the type of stationary phase applied to the plate. The method is rapid, taking as little as an hour as compared to 7-8 hrs of PC. Compounds can be detected in a much lower concentration as the spots are very compact. Separated compounds can be detected by corrosive sprays and elevated temperature e.g. spraying with 50% sulphuric acid or 25% sulphuric acid in ethanol and heating will result in most compounds becoming charred and showing up as brown spots. This is not possible with paper which will burn and disintegrate.

5. SAMPLE COLLECTION, PRESERVATION AND PREPARATION

These are identical for all chromatographic methods as for any other biochemical investigation of biological fluids or tissues. The complex mixtures of substances present in biological fluids often results in their mutual interference when chromatography of a particular group of compounds is being attempted. Either the interferences must be removed or the substances of interest selectively extracted. Care must be taken at this

stage to prevent or at least minimise losses. Sometimes substances are converted to more satisfactory derivatives which are subsequently chromatographed eg labile keto-acids are converted to stable di-nitrophenyl hydrazones or amino acids which may be separated by TLC or PC.

6. ADSORPTION CHROMATOGRAPHY

6.1. Principle

Separation of components of a mixture depends on differences both in their degree of adsorption and solubility in the solvent used for separation. This can be carried out in the Column, Thin-layer and Paper mode. Compounds are adsorbed onto the stationary phase to an extent determined by the charge, van der Waal's forces, dipole interactions, hydrogen bonding and steric factors. This depends on the structure of the components due to which they have greater or lesser affinity for the stationary and mobile phases.

The mass of solute adsorbed per unit weight of adsorbent (m) depends on the concentration of the solute (c) and Langmuir derived an equation on the basis that (a) only a monolayer is adsorbed (b) Only a proportion of the molecules in collision will get adsorbed. This is known as Langmuir adsorption isotherm.

$$m = \frac{k_1\, k_2 c}{1 + k_2\, c}$$

K_1 is a measure of the number of active adsorption sites per unit weight of adsorbent and depends on the nature of the adsorbent. K_2 is a measure of the affinity of solute for the adsorbent and is affected by all the components of the system.

Langmuir assumed only one binding site, but in practice there are a number of binding sites on the surface of the adsorbent each with a different affinity, thus giving a series of Langmuir type isotherms. Hinshelwood therefore suggested that the equation.

$$m = \frac{k_1\, k_2\, c}{1 + k_2\, c}$$

gives a more accurate picture. This approximates to Freundlich adsorption isotherm found in practice.

$$m = K c^x$$

K and x are constants depending on the particular system used.

The difference between these two isotherms is illustrated in the graph (Fig. 2.7a)

The mixture of binding sites of different affinities is the cause of tailing observed in the elution profile in Column Chromatography (Fig. 2.7b). This tailing can be overcome by eluting with a suitable gradient of pH, ionic strength or polarity so that the more strongly adsorbed molecules meet a higher concentration of displacing compound than the more weakly bound molecules.

Adsorbents

Compounds such as silicic acid (silica gel), aluminium oxide, $CaCO_3$, $MgCO_3$, $ZnCO_3$, MgO & cellulose may be used as stationary phase. The choice of any adsorbent and solvent depends on the separation to be achieved. Hydroxyapetite ($CaPO_4$) is widely used for the separation of proteins, nucleic acids and viruses. Unlike most other adsorbents it has some ion-exchange properties which aids separation. In addition, in nucleic acid

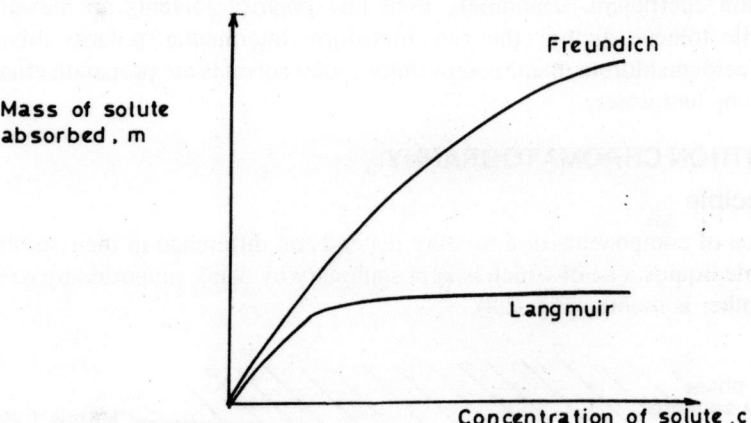

Fig. 2.7 (a) : Adsorption isotherms of freundlich and langmuir

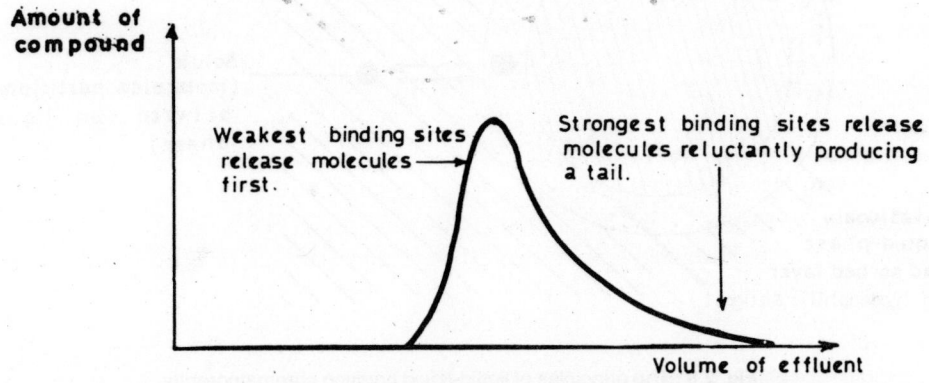

Fig. 2.7 (b) : Tailing observed in the flution of a compound from an adsorption column.

separation it has the advantage that it can bind to double-stranded DNA but not single-stranded DNA. Adsorbents of TLC are often impregnated with $AgNO_3$ to enhance separation of compounds differing in the number of double bonds. This is called argentation TLC. Some adsorbents have a tendency to take up water from the atmosphere during storage and this may adversely affect their adsorption properties. In such cases, the adsorbents are activated by heating at 110C for some time to remove any water.

Poly-E-caprolactam TLC sheets do not require activation and are semi- transparent allowing unknowns and standards to run on opposite sides to be compared. They cam be reused if immediately cleared with ammonia- acetone and are widely used in protein sequencing. In general, the adsorption affinity of compounds increases with polarity of molecules, with the number of double bonds in alkenes and with the introduction of functional groups. In order of increasing affinity some functional groups are as follows:

—O —R, —NO_2, —COR, —OCOR, —NH_2, —OH, — $CONH_2$, —COOH

6.3 Solvents

The choice depends upon the polarity of the compounds to be resolved and upon their distribution coefficient. Commonly used low polarity solvents are hexane, heptane, acetonitrile, toluene, diethyl ether and chloroform. Intermediate polarity solvents include ethanoic acid, dichloromethane and pyridine, polar solvents are propanol, ethanol, methanol, acetone and water.

7. PARTITION CHROMATOGRAPHY

7.1 Principle

Separation of components of a mixture depends on difference in their solubility in two immiscible liquids, one of which is kept stationary by being supported by an inert matrix and the other is mobile (Fig. 2.8).

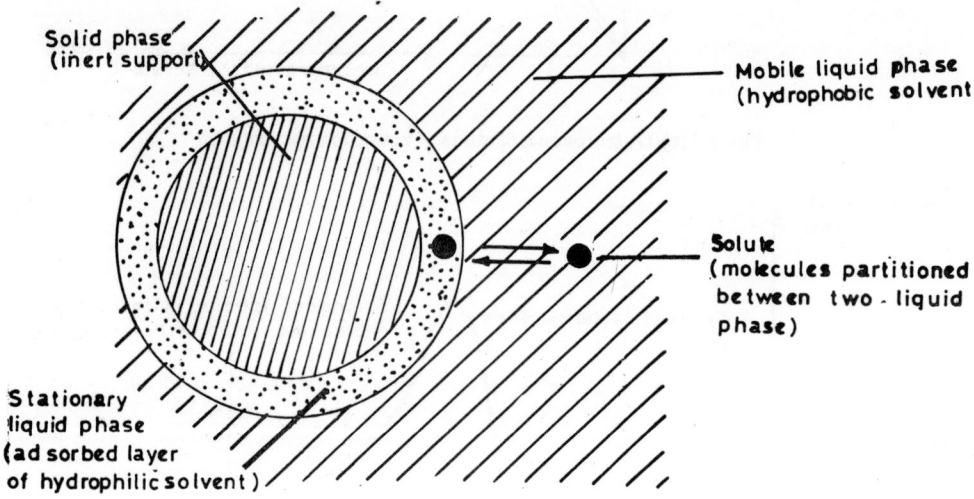

Fig. 2.8 : The principles of liquid-liquid partition chromatography.

The component distributes itself between the two immiscible liquid phases as described by the partition coefficient K_d at equilibrium. As already mentioned

$$K_d = \frac{\text{Concentration in solvent 1}}{\text{Concentration in solvent 2}}$$

In Normal Phase Partition Chromatography the stationary phase is usually water while the mobile phase is an organic non polar liquid, immiscible in water that flows past the stationary phase. Thus compounds, that are soluble in both water and non-polar organic solvents are readily separated by partition methods, as compared to adsorption chromatography in which compounds sparingly soluble in water but insoluble in organic liquids are separated.

In case of column chromatography the matrix may be cellulose starch or silicic acid, for TLC it is most commonly cellulose, whereas for paper partition chromatography sufficient water is naturally present in paper to act as stationary phase.

In Reverse Phase Partition Chromatography the stationary phase is a non-polar liquid e.g. liquid paraffin supported by an inert matrix as in normal phase.This phase is prepared by treating the supporting matrix with a solution of the mobile phase in a suitable non-polar and volatile solvent the solvent is subsequently removed by evaporation.

7.1 Counter Current Chromatography

Counter Current Chromatography (CCC) is a separation process based on distribution of a compound between two immiscible liquid phases but neither phase is supported on an inert matrix. In this it differs from conventional liquid-liquid partition chromatography. The mixture components are partitioned between two immiscible liquid phases which move relative to one another. The usual form of apparatus comprises a series of extraction tubes through which the less dense of the two phases moves. Each extraction is performed by shaking the tubes and, after a period to allow the phases to separate, transfer of the upper phase is effected. The components of the mixture progress through the tubes as a result of the movement of phases but at different rates. These rates depend on the K of the components in the two phases, when these coefficients are different separation is achieved.

7.3. High Performance Liquid Chromatography (HPLC)

7.3.1. Principle

HPLC is a form of chromatography in the column mode, using small particle size stationary phase and high pressure eluant pumping systems to give a high performance hence High Performance Liquid Chromatography.

All forms of column Chromatography rely on gravity or low pressure pumping systems for supply of eluant to the column. The flow rates are therefore low and cannot be increased by merely increasing the pressure of the eluant supply as this would create a back pressure which would eventually damage the column structure. The use of smaller particle size stationary phases make it possible to withstand these high pressures and, at the same time give better resolutions since the total surface area and therefore the number of binding sites increases unfortunately, smaller particle size offers greater resistance to eluant flow. In recent years, however, special pumping systems have been designed which can give higher flow rates. These, together with the use of small particle size stationary phase result in quick, efficient and better resolution in adsorption, partition, ion exchange, exclusion and affinity column chromatography. Hence, this is called high performance liquid chromatography (HPLC).

The principal components of an HPLC system are shown in Fig. 2.9.

7.3.2 The Column

Columns are generally made of stainless steel and are manufactured such that they can withstand pressures upto 5.5×10 Pa (8000 p.s.i) straight columns of 20cm - 50cm length, 1-4 mmm diameter with an internal mirror finish to allow efficient packing of columns are used. Porous plugs of stainless steel or teflon are used at the base of the columns to retain the packing material. The plugs must be homogenous to ensure uniform flow of solvent through the column. In some separations it is required to maintain constant temperature. This is thermostatically controlled.

7.3.3. Column Packing

Three forms of column packing material are available:

(1) Microporous supports where micropores ramify through the particles which are 5-10 µm in diameter.

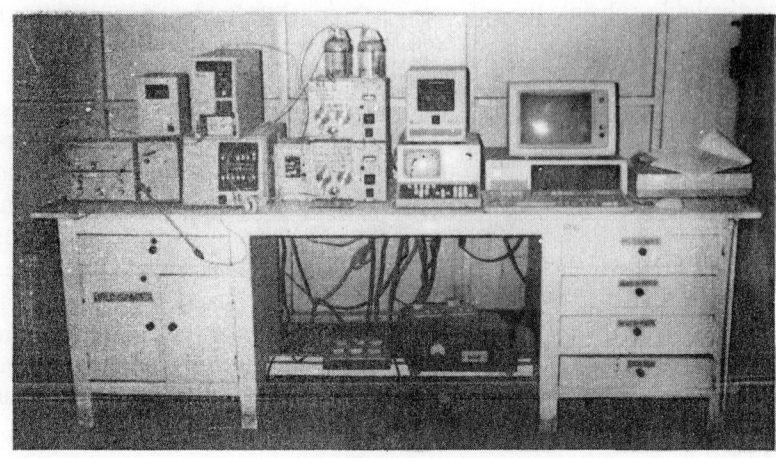

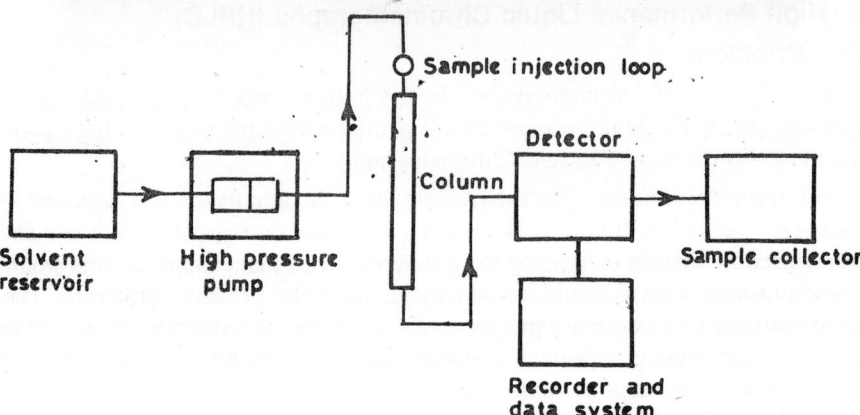

Fig. 2.9 : Diagrammatic representation of the components of an isocartic HPLC system (Inset) an HPLC column with associated pumps, detector and recording instruments.

(2) Pellicular supports where porous particles are coated onto an inert solid core such as a glass bead of about 40 μm in diameter.

(3) Bonded phases where the stationary phase is chemically bonded onto an inert support.

For adsorption chromatography, adsorbents such as silica or alumina are available as microporous or pellicular forms with a range of particle sizes. Pellicular forms have a high efficiency but low sample capacity and therefore microporous supports are prefered where applicable. All HPLC packing materials are regular, spherical in shape giving good packing and flow properties.

In liquid - liquid partition systems the stationary phase may be coated onto an inert support. Both microporous and pellicular supports are used, but in these the stationary solvent gradually gets washed out with the mobile solvent. To overcome this, bonded phases have been developed. Where the stationary liquid is covalently bonded to the supporting material which may be silica or a silicone polymer.

Many different types of ion exchangers are available of which the cross - linked microporous polystyrene resins are widely used. Pellicular resin forms are also available, as are bonded phase exchangers covalently bonded to a cross linked silicone network. These are called hard gels and readily withstand pressures required during analysis.

The stationary phases for exclusion chromatography in the HPLC mode are porous silica, glass, polystyrene or polyvinylacetate beads. These are generally used with organic eluting solvents semirigid gels such as sephadex and non rigid gels such as sepharose are or of limited use in HPLC since they can withstand only low pressures. The supports for affinity separations are same as those for exclusion apparatus. The spacer arm and ligand are chemically bound to the support.

Column Packing Procedure

The most widely used is the high pressure slurrying technique. A suspension of the packing is made in a solvent of equal density to the packing material. The slurry is then rapidly pumped at high pressure into a column with a porous plug at its outlet. The resulting bed of packing material can then be prepared for used by running the mobile phase through the column when hard gels are packed, it is necessary to allow them to swell first in the solvent to be used in the chromatographic separation before packing under pressure. Soft gels cannot be packed under pressure and are allowed to pack from a slurry, in the column under gravitational sedimentation only, as in conventional column chromatography.

7.3.4. Chromatographic Solvent (mobile phase)

The choice of mobile phase depends on the type of separation to be achieved. Isocratic separations may be made using a single solvent, or two solvents or more solvents mixed in fixed proportions. Alternatively gradient elution system may be used. For this two pumps are required to pump the two solvents to produce a gradient. In all cases, the solvent should be free of even traces of impurities as this would hamper the development and interfere in the detection of compounds. To this end, 1-5 μm microfilters are attached prior to the pump even though extra pure, HPLC solvents are commercially available.

7.3.5. Pumping Systems

The main features of a good pumping system is that it should be capable of outputs of at least 3.4 x 10^7 Pa (5000 psi) and there should be no pulses of flow through the sytem. There must be a flow delivery of at least 10 cm   min   for normal analysis and upto 30 cm min for preparative analysis . Several pumping systems are available which operate on the principle of constant pressure or constant displacement. Constant pressure pumps produce a pulseless flow through the column, but any decrease in the permeability of the column will result in lower flow rates for which the pump will not compensate. These pumps operate by the introduction of high pressure gas into the pump and the gas in turn forces the solvent from the pump chamber into the column. The use of an intermediate solvent between the gas and the eluting solvent reduces the chances of dissolved gas directly entering the eluting solvent and causing problems during analysis.

Constant displacement pumps maintain a constant flow rate through the column irrespective of changing conditions within the column. One form of constant displacement pump is a motor driven syringe type. Pump where a fixed volume of solvent is forced from the pump to the column by a piston driven by a motor. Such pumps provide uniform solvent flow rates and also yield a pulseless solvent flow which is important as certain detectors are sensitive to changes in solvent flow rate.

7.3.6. Detector Systems

Most commonly the detector is a variable wavelength UV spectrophotometer, fluorimeter, refractive index monitor or an electrochemical detector. A recent development is the interfacing of HPLC to a mass spectrometer. In all cases the detector should be very sensitive since the quantity of material is very small.

7.3.7. Practical Procedure

The correct application of a sample onto a HPLC column is important in achieving successful separations. Ideally, the sample should be introduced as an infinitely narrow band into the column. Two methods are generally used. The first method makes use of microsyringe designed to withstand high pressure. The sample is injected through a system in an injection port, either directly onto the column packing or onto a small plug of inert material immediately above the column packing.

The second method is by the use of a loop injector. This consists of a metal loop of small volume which can be filled with the sample by means of an appropriate valve, the eluant from the pump is channeled through the loop, the outlet of which leads to the column. The sample is thus flushed onto the column by the eluant, without interruption of solvent flow to the column. Automatic versions of loop injectors are commercially available.

8. GAS LIQUID CHROMATOGRAPHY

8.1. Principle

The difference in partition coefficient of volatalised components of a mixture, between a stationary liquid and mobile gas phases as the compounds are carried through the column by the mobile gas phase. As the compounds leave the column they pass through a detector which is linked via an amplifier to a chart recorder which in turn records a peak as a compound passes through the detector (Fig. 2.10)

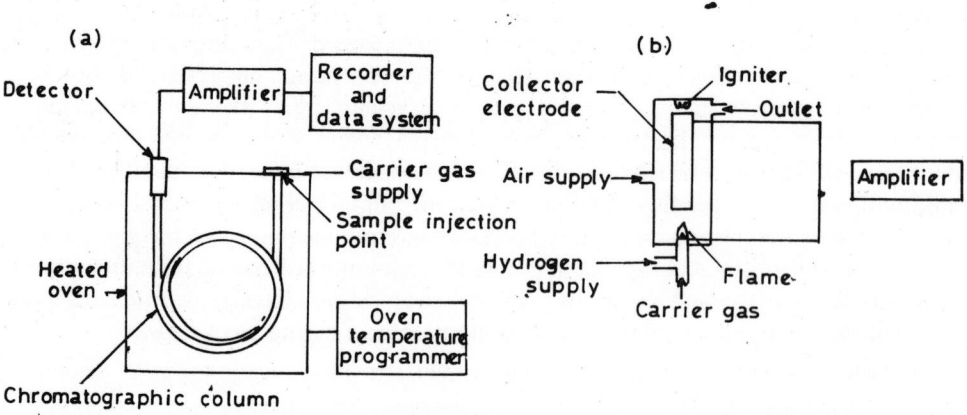

Fig. 2.10 : Diagrammatic representation of (a) GLC system and (b) Flame ionisation detector.

This can be carried out only in the column mode. It has high sensitivity, reproducibility and speed of resolution and has proved to be the most versatile of all chromatographic methods. The only limiting factor is that the components of the mixture must be vaporised to give heat stable vapours upto a temperature of 300 C.

8.2. Apparatus and Materials

The mobile gas phase known as the carrier gas has to be chemically inert. N , Ar and He are used. The mixture to be separated is introduced as a liquid to the stream of carrier gas through an injection device where it vaporises and passes into the column containing the stationary liquid phase despersed on an inert supporting solid. The column is in an oven whose temperature can be precisely regulated. Separation takes place during passage through the column and components of the mixture emerge in well separated zones. The outlet from the column passes through the detector which analyses the gas stream and indicates via a pen recorder the emergence of each component (Fig. 2.11).

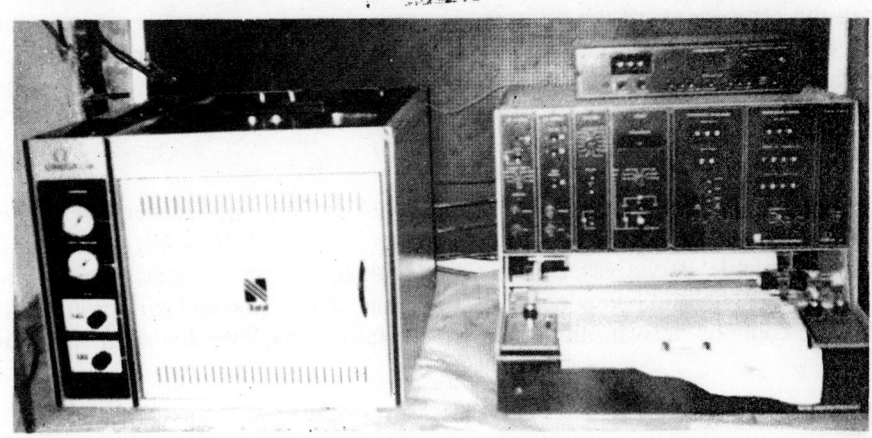

. (Inset) A gas liquid chromatograph on the left with detector and recorder on the right.

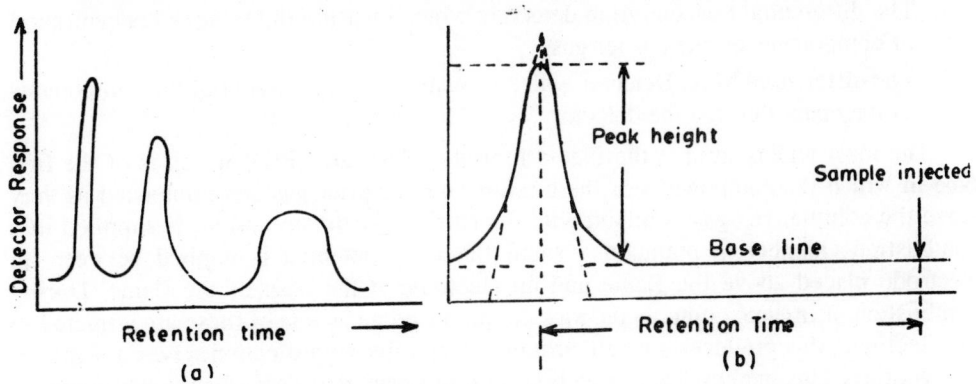

Fig. 2.11 (a) : Schematic recorder trace from a gas-liquid chromatograph (b) An idealised gas-liquid recorder peak showing the significance of retention time.

Under a given set of operating conditions a particular compound is always eluted at a definite retention time (tr) which corresponds to a definite volume of gas passed called retention volume (Vr). The identification of a component is made by comparing the retention time of a peak in a mixture with that obtained from a pure compound under identical conditions.

The solid support on which the stationary liquid phase is dispersed should be inert to the sample. It is usually calcite (diatomaceous silica) celite is often silanised with hexamethyldisilazane so that its reactive hydroxyl groups are modified. The support particles have an even size of 60 to 80, 80 to 100 or 100 to 120 mesh size which is a measure of the openings per inch in a sieve hence the larger mesh size is, smaller the particle is.

The stationary phase should be chemically unreactive with sample. It should also be thermally stable at the high temperature used for analysis. If it is not thermally stable, it volatalises. This votalisation called "column bleed" contaminates the detector giving an unstable baseline. The general rule for selecting the liquid phase is that it should be similar to the components of the mixture. Thus the separation of hydrocarbons is best achieved on a non polar stationary phase such as squaline. While separation of esters takes place most efficiently on a more polar liquid such as polyethylene glycol adipate a polyester.

8.3. Preparation and Injection of Sample

The majority of non and low polar compounds are directly applied because of their volatility. Other compounds possessing polar groups such as —OH, —NH, —COOH are converted to volatile dervatives before GLC analysis. These includes amino acids, carbohydrates, nucleic acid components. Methylation, silanisation and trifluoromethylsilanisation are common derivatisation methods for fatty acids, carbohydrates and amino acids.

8.4. Detection Systems

There are several methods used for detecting the presence of compounds in the outlet carrier gas stream. These fall into two basic types:

1. The differential concentration detectors which measure the relative concentration of components on the carrier gas.
2. The differential Mass Detector which measure absolute amount of the components as they pass through the detector.

The most widely used is the Flame Ionisation Detector (FID) which is of the first type in which the components of the mixture in the carrier gas are combusted as they leave the column. H_2 gas is mixed with the carrier gas stream and air is supplied in a combustion chamber to maintain a small flame. A potential is applied between an electrode placed above the flame and an electrode at the base of the flame. During combustion of organic compounds, ions are produced and some of these are attracted to the electrode, this produces a small current, which after amplification, gives a signal to the recorder. This method has a detection limit of about 10^{-12}g s^{-1} and an upper temperature limit of 400° C.

The Thermal Conductivity Detector (TCD) or Katharometer detector measures the change in thermal conductivity of the carrier gas as a component emerges. This is measured by means of change in resistance of a platinum wire. All components of a mixture whether organic or inorganic are detected upto a limit of 10^{-8}g s^{-1}.

The Nitrogen Phosphorous Detector (NPD) also called thermionic detector is similar in design to FID but has a sodium salt fused onto the electrode system or a burner tip embedded in a ceramic tube containing a sodium salt or a rubidium chloride tip. It gives a good response towards N and P containing compounds. Its detection limit 10^{-11} g s^{-1} g s and upper temperature limit of 300°C do not compare well with FID. Nevertheless this is widely used in organophosphorous pesticide residue analysis.

The Electron Capture Detector (ECD) responds only to substances which capture electrons e.g. halogen containing compounds. It works by means of a radioactive source (63_{Ni}) ionising the column gas and the electrons so produced give a current across the electrodes to which a suitable voltage is applied. When an electron capturing compound emerges from the column the ionised electrons are captured, the current drops and this change in current is recorded. The carrier gas used in conjunction with an ECD is N or Ar + 5 % methane mixture. It has a detection limit of 10^{12} g s-1, upper temperature limit of 300 C and is particularly useful in the analysis of polychlorinated compounds like pesticides e.g. DDT, dieldrin, aldrin.

These detectors respond variably to the volatile solvent used to inject the mixture and give a solvent peak at the beginning of the chromatogram.

In cases where identity of a compound is unknown the GLC is connected to a mass spectrometer. Special separators separate the carrier gas from the sample which is introduced into the mass spectrometer. The GLC can also be linked to IR spectrometer and NMR spectrometer in order to identify the compounds.

9. ION EXCHANGE CHROMATOGRAPHY

9.1. Principle

As different from other forms of chromatography, ion-exchange chromatography depends on the degree of attraction between oppositely charged particles. Hence this is used exclusively for the separation of ionic species. These occur mainly in inorganic systems. However, in organic systems too, amino acids, proteins and nucleic acids components have ionisable groups which can carry positive or negative charge depending on their pKa and pH of the solution. Separation may be carried out in the column, paper or thin layer modes with the help of ion exchanges which are materials positively charged groups (anion exchangers) or negatively charged groups (cation exchangers). The positive and negative charges in the exchangers are loosely bound to oppositely charged groups. When a group of stronger charge is introduced into the matrix structure of the exchanges, they displace the loosely bound groups and themselves bind strongly as a result of higher degree of attraction eg:

$$RSO_3^- \ldots Na^+ \quad + \quad N^+H_3R' \quad = \quad RSO_3^- \ldots NH_3R' + Na^+$$

Cation exchanger : exchanger counter   charged   bound molecular excha-
                 ion   molecule   ion   nged
                to be excha-   ion
                    nged

Anion Exchanger: $(R)_4N^+ \ldots Cl^-$ + $OOCR =$ $(R)_4 N^+ \ldots OOCR' + Cl$

The exchanged molecules are recovered by selective desorption by the eluant and diffusion of the molecule to the external solution. Selective disorption is brought about by changing pH, ionic concentration or by introducing an ion which has greater affinity for the exchanger than the bound molecules.

9.2. Materials

The common ion exchange materials are resins insoluble in water. These are made by copolymeresation of styrene and divinyl benzene. Copolymerisation results in cross linkages which renders the polymers insoluble by varying the amount of the two polymers the amount of cross linking is controlled so that the system swells in water and is successible to water molecules and ionic species. Sulphonic acid groups are introduced after polymerisation. This provides the anionic group which binds mobile cations-cation exchanger (Fig. 2.12) Anion exchangers are made by copolymerising styrene with chlormethyl ether and then reacting the chloro groups with tertiary amines which provides the cationic group which binds mobile anions . Anion exchanger. As an alternative to polystyrene based exchangers, modified celluloses are now available which posseses good flow and exchange properties. In addition, separation is aided by the sieving action of gels and beads of these materials.

10. EXCLUSION CHROMATOGRAPHY

10.1. Principle

Separation of molecules on the basis of their molecular size and shape utilising the molecular sieve action of gels. The term gel filtration is used to describe the separation of molecules of varying molecular size utilizing the gel materials. Porous glass granules have been used for this purpose and the term controlled pore glass chromatography coined for this process. The term exclusion or permeation chromatography is used to describe all separation processes utilising the molecular sieve action of gels.

Gels are insoluble hydrophilic semi-solid colloids which swell in buffer to form a 3-dimensional network of pores. In order to explain the molecular sieve action of gels, consider a mixture of large, medium and small particles being eluted through a gel (in equilibrium with a suitable solvent for the molecules to be separated.)

Large molecules which are completely excluded from the pores of the gel particles will pass through the interstitial spaces first, while small molecules wil be distributed between the solvent inside and outside the gel particles and will then pass through the column at a slower rate. Due to variation in the pore size of gel particles, molecules of medium size will penetrate either partially, fully or not at all (Fig 2.13b). Hence, the distribution coefficient K_d of a particular solute between inner and outer solvent of a particular gel system will vary between $K_d = 0$, for large molecules completely excluded, to $K_d = 1$ for small particles which completely reach the inner solvent. The intermediate values will be for molecules of medium size. These variable K values are responsible for the complete separation of components of a mixture based on differences in molecular weight or size.

The elution volume for a given solute depends on several parameters given by the expression:

$$Ve = Vo + K_d\, Vi$$

(1)

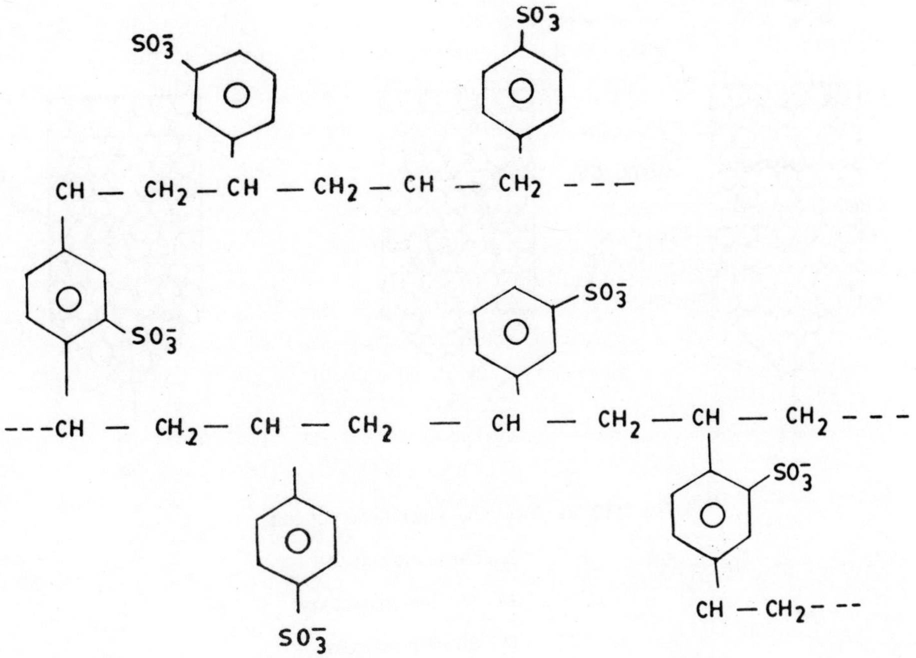

SULPHONATED POLYSTYRENE RESIN

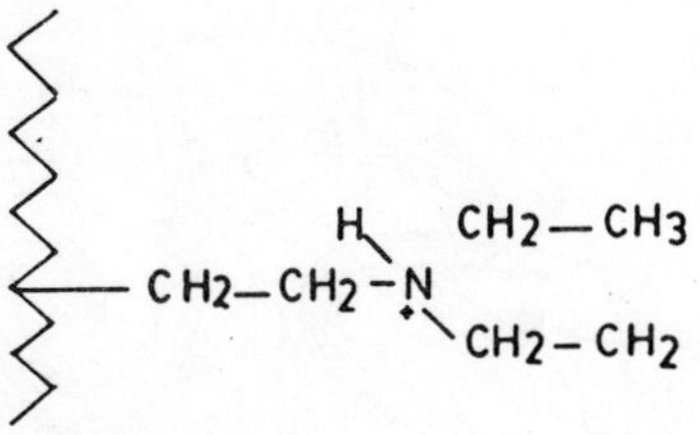

CELLULOSE
DEAE CELLULOSE
(DIETHYLAMINOETHYL CELLULOSE)

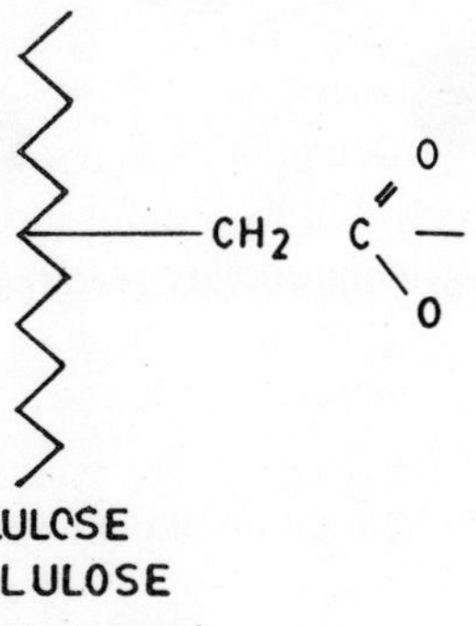

CELLULOSE
C M CELLULOSE
(CARLOXYMETAYLCELLULOSE)

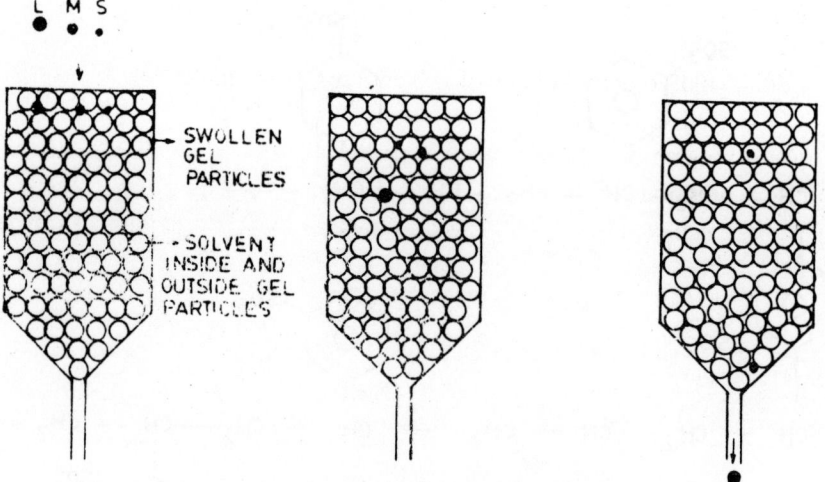

Fig. 2.13 (a) : Molecular sieve action of gels

L = Large molecules

M = Medium molecules

, S = Small moolecules

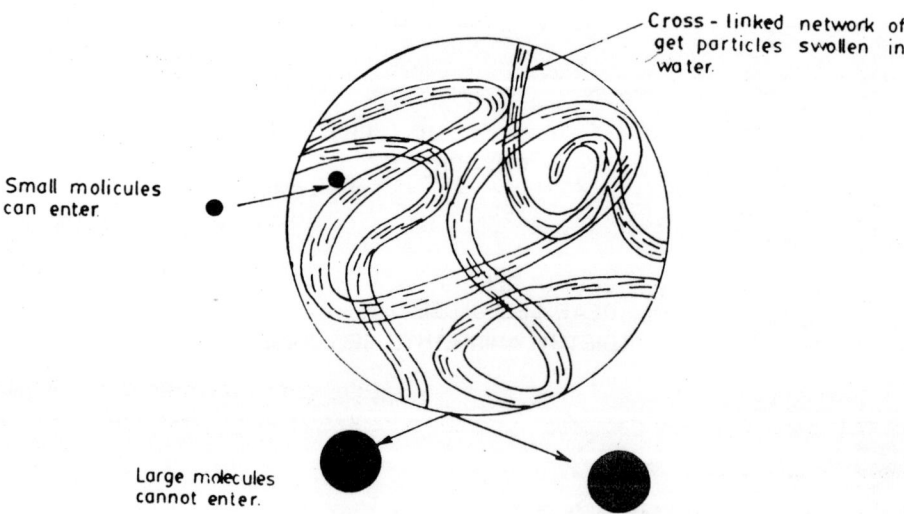

Fig. 2.13 (b) : The Principle of Gel Filtration

where,

Vo = void volume (volume of solvent outside gel particles)

Ve = elution volume

Vi = volume of solvent inside gel particles

K_d = partition coefficient

Vi can be calculated from Wr, water regain value, that is the amount of solvent taken up by 1g of dry gel.

$$Vi = aWr \qquad (2)$$

a = dry weight of gel.

Thus from (1)

$$K_d = \frac{Ve - Vo}{Vi} = \frac{Ve - Vo}{aWr}$$

For a molecular species completely exclude Ve = Vo

$$K_d = O$$

Fig. 2.14 shows the elution diagram for exclusion chromatography.

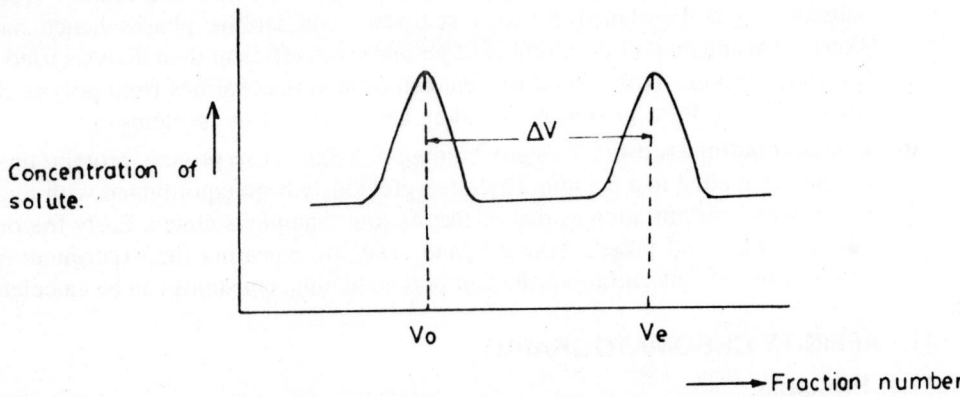

Fig. 2.14 : Elution Diagram for exclusion chromatography.

The molecular weight of a given unknown species can be determined by comparing its Δ V value with that of compounds of known molecular weight eluted under the same conditions.

10.2. Materials and Methods

Gel filtration is carried out in the column mode usually. However, thin layer mode can also be employed. The swollen gel is spread onto the glass plate without the addition of a binding material. This is called Thin Layer Gel Filtration (TLG) like TLC the solvent in the interstitial spaces is the mobile phase but unlike it, the layer is never dried hence there is no solvent front. The plate is kept in an air tight jar at an angle of 20 to the horizontal to facilitate movement of solvent through the layer. While TLC is used for separation of amino acids, sugars, oligosaccharides and lipophilic substances. TLG is used for separation of hydrophilic substances particularly high molecular weight biological material like proteins, nucleic acids etc.

10.3 Applications

Apart from the use of the method for separation of components of a mixture, gel filtration has further uses not found in any other chromatographic technique. These include:

(a) Determination of molecular weight of an unknown compound
(b) Concentration of solute
(c) Desalting of proteins
(d) Protein binding studies.

(a) **Determination of molecular weight of an unknown compound :** For determination of molecular weight of an unknown compound, V (Ve - Vo) values are compared with Δ V values of known compounds eluted under the same conditions.

(b) **Concentration of solute :** Water and low molecular weight substances are absorbed by the swelling gel while high molecular weight substances remain in solution. After 10 minutes gel is removed by centrifugation leaving high molecular weight material in a solution whose concentration has increased without altering pH and ionic strength.

(c) **Desalting solutions of high molecular weight compounds :** High molecular weight substances move with the void volume while low molecular weight substances get distributed between stationary and mobile phases hence move slowly. This method of desalting is faster and more efficient than dialysis used for the same purpose. This is used for removal of monosaccharides from polysaccharides, NH_4 SO_4 from protein preparation, amino acids from proteins etc.

(d) **Protein binding studies :** To study binding of a ligand to a protein, protein/ ligand mixture is applied to a column which has previously been equilibrated with ligand of the same concentration as that of the mixture. Sample is eluted. Early fractions contain ligand and protein bound ligand. Thus by repeating the experiment at a series of ligand concentrations the appropriate binding constants can be calculated.

11. AFFINITY CHROMATOGRAPHY

11.1. Principle

Unlike all other separation and preparative techniques like chromatography, centrifugation, electrophoresis which depend on physical properties (size, molecular weight) of molecules, affinity chromatograph depends on biological interactions of molecules to achieve purification. It is therefore very sensitive and extremely efficient in achieving absolute purity in a single process without destruction of the molecules. This factor makes it superior from other forms of chromatography where repeated fractionation is necessary to achieve a high degree of purity.

It is well known that an enzyme can bind specifically to substrate, inhibiter or activator. These are called ligands.

A column is prepared in which a ligand of the required enzyme is covalently bonded to the inert insoluble matrix when a solution containing the enzyme is passed through this column, it alone binds to the ligand while all other molecules pass through. Even slightly modified or denatured molecules do not bind and are thus eliminated. The enzyme is then eluted by either changing the pH or ionic srength of solvent. Originally, the technique was developed for the purification of enzymes but it has now been extended to nucleotides, nucleic acids, immunoglobulins, membrane receptors and even whole cells and cell fragments, that is any molecule capable of reversibily binding to a specific ligand which is attached to an insoluble matrix.

$$M \quad + \quad L \quad \underline{K_{+1}} \quad M\,L$$

Macromolecule   Ligand K_{-1} Complex

The main limitation found so far is that of simulating the natural affinity between macromolecules in an artificial system. It requires detailed knowledge of such interactions and conditions (pH, ionic strength, temperature etc.) in which these can take place. Also, the matrix in which the ligand is bound should have spherical gel particles for good flow of the unbound molecules to pass through. Further, the ligand should be attached such that the attachment site for the macromolecule is well exposed. For this reason the ligand is not bound directly to the matrix, instead, a spacer arm, is used to separate the two (Fig. 2.15)

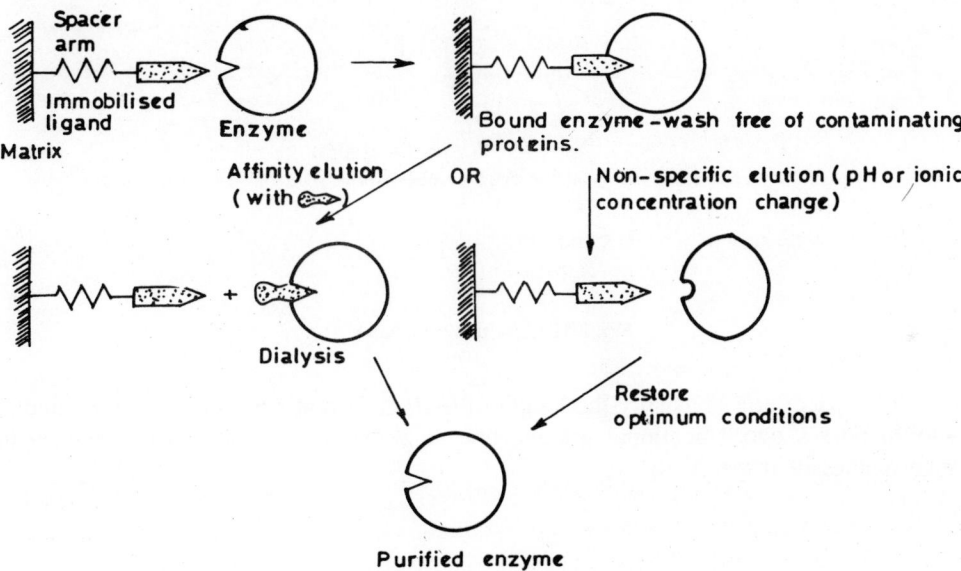

Fig. 2.15 : Diagrammatic representation of purification of an enzyme by affinity chromatography.

11.2. Materials and Methods

The three important components of an affinity chromatograph are the matrix, ligand and spacer arm.

The matrix should have a good network of pores through which unbound molecules can easily pass. It should be inert chemically and should have suitable functional groups to which the ligand can bind. It should not interact or interact only weakly with other molecules so that non- specific adsorption does not occur. The most commonly used materials are agarose and polyacrylamide gels, cellulose, porous glass and silica.

Ligands may be bonded to the matrix with the aid of cyanogen bromide treatment of matrix at pH 11 (Fig. 2.16) which activates the matrix for ligand attachment.

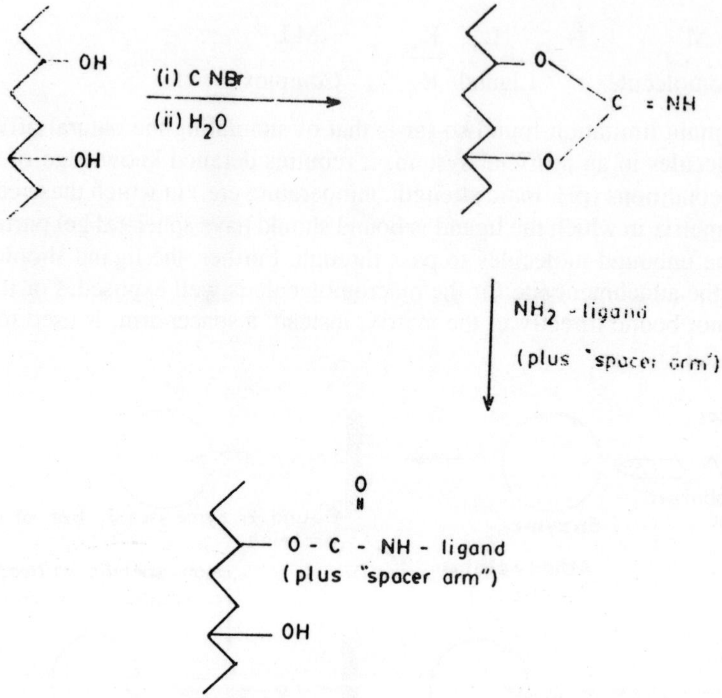

Fig. 2.16 : The use of "Spacer Arm"

The spacer arm is usually the length of 6-10 carbon atoms or their equivalent. It should posses two functional groups, one at either end to bind to the matrix and macromolecule respectively.

3

SPECTROSCOPY

1. INTRODUCTION

1.1 Definition and General Principles

As a useful working definition spectroscopy can be defined as the interaction of electromagnetic radiation with matter, although this does not include mass spectroscopy. Several factors have led to the branching of spectroscopy in different directions. Most significant is the order of magnitude of energies involved, but additional factors eg presence of a magnetic field and instrumentation considerations have led to the techniques of UV, IR, NMR, ESR spectroscopy.

Break-up and analysis of the above definition will be useful before delving into the details of the different spectroscopic techniques already mentioned.

The definition includes

   (i) Electromagnetic Radiation

  (ii) Interaction of electromagnetic radiation with matter

 (iii) Matter

Electromagnetic radiation consists of an electric field parpendecular to a magnetic field and both at right angles to the direction of propagation of light (Fig. 3.1) A fundamental property of electromagnetic radiation is that it can behave as though it exists as discrete quanta or packets of energy.

$E = h\nu$

where,

    E = energy

    h = Planck's constant = 6.63×10^{-34} Js

    ν = frequsency of radiation in Hertz

There are two ways in which EM radiation interacts with matter viz. absorption and emission. Absorption occurs when incident radiation increases the energy of a system.

Increase in energy is manifested as a decrease in intensity of emergent radiation. Emission occurs when there is a decrease in the energy of a system. Decrease in energy may be manifested is :

    (1) Thermal energy loss : energy loss by molecular or sub molecular motion like

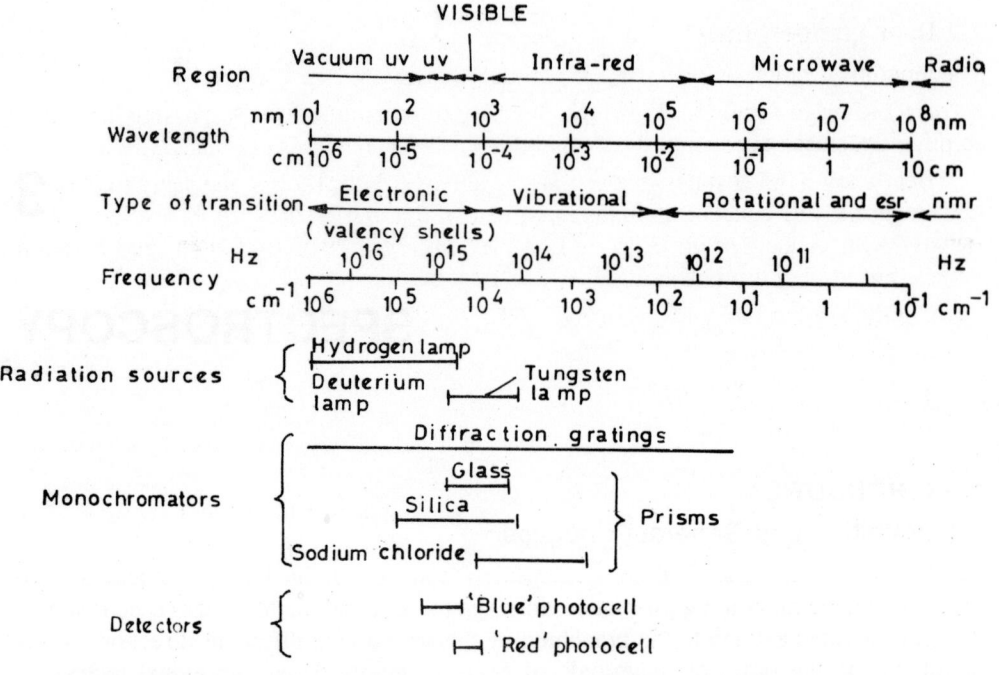

Fig. 3.1 : The electromagnetic spectrum and spectral characteristics of spectrophotometer. Components.

collision, vibration and rotation.

(2) Electromagnetic emission : this results in phosphorescence and fluorescence.

(3) Photochemical reactions : there is a competition between the three processes also called relaxation processes.

Matter is composed of atoms and molecules. The electrons are constrained to certain energy levels called K L M etc. orbitals. When atoms combine to form molecules electrons occupy new energy levels called Molecular Bonding Orbitals. Atoms in the molecule can vibrate and rotate about the bond axis giving rise to vibrational and rotational energy sublevels. Electrons usually remain in the ground state but on receiving energy e.g. from incident electromagnetic radiation, get excited to higher states. This is absorption of energy. When electrons come back to the original ground state, emission of energy takes place. Sometimes all the energy absorbed is emitted while at other times some energy is lost in one or all of the relaxation processes. The amount of energy absorbed or emitted is given by

$$E = E_1 - E_2 = h$$

where, E_1 = energy of electron at original level

E_2 = energy of electron at final level

h = Planck's constant = 6.63×10^{-34} Js

c = Velocity of light = 3×10 ms^{-1}

v = Frequency of radiation in Hertz = C/λ

λ = Wavelength of radiation usually in nanometers

1.2 Beer Lambert Law

The amount of radiation absorbed or emitted is given by Beer-Lambert Law.

According to Lambert (1760) the intensity of transmitted   light passing through a solution decreases exponentially as thickness of layer increases arithmetically.

Beer's law (1852) states that each molecule of solute absorbs the same fraction of light regardless of concentration. That is to say, that the absorbance of a solute varies linearly with concentration (Fig. 3.2). It does not hold good over high concentration ranges, but in very dilute solutions.

Combining the two laws we arrive at the Beer Lambert law given by

$$I = I_o \ 10^{-\varepsilon cl}$$

where

    I = intensity of incident beam of monochromatic light passing through an absorbing species

    I_o = intensity of emergent radiation which is less than incident intensity.

      = Molar absorptivity constant at that wavelength

    c = concentration of the absorbing species in mol/l l = optical path length usually 1 cm.

Taking log

    $\log \ I/ Io \ = - \varepsilon cl \ \log_{10}$

    $\log = Io/ I \ = \ \varepsilon cl$

    since $\log Io/ I = A$ (absorbance)

    $A = \ \varepsilon cl$

The ratio I/I_o is called transmittance, T and hence

    $- \log T = A$

When T is measured as a percentage, it is related to A mathematically as follows:

    $A = 2.0 - \log \% \ T$

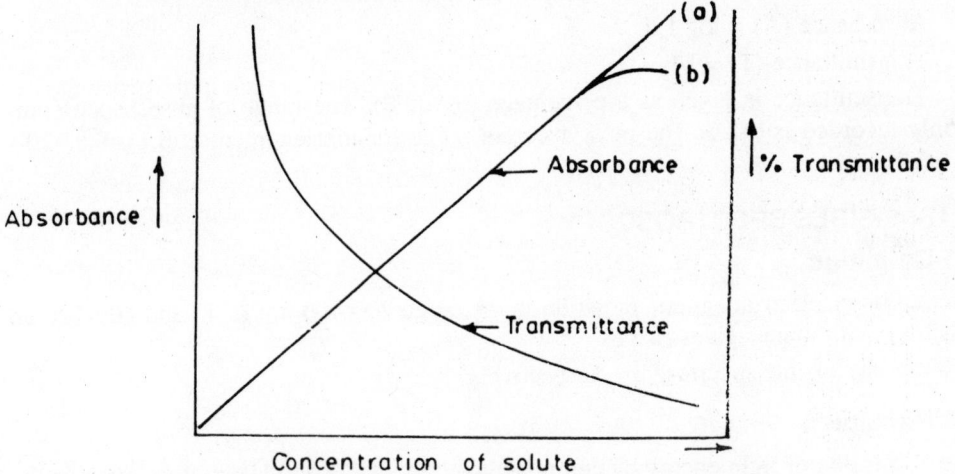

Fig. 3.2 (a) : Beer's law plot **(b)** Deviation from Beer's law

A spectrum is a plot of absorption or emission versus wavelength. The spectra of atoms are line spectra since the electrons are present in discrete energy levels. In molecules also electrons are present in discrete energy levels. However, a group of molecules exists in a number of different vibrational and rotational states, each state differing from another by a relatively small amount of energy. Thus a group of molecules absorbs energy over a small range to give rise to an absorption band over certain ranges of wavelength, the absorbance rises to a maximum and the transmittance falls to a minimum (Fig. 3.3). This is referred to as an absorption peak.

In quantitative analysis the values of absorption peak are used so that measurement have greatest sensitivity with respect to solute concentration. Also, the value obtained is least sensitive to errors in wavelength setting of the spectrophotometer.

1.3 Mechanics of Measurement

The basic requirements of a spectrophotometer are as follows :

(a) Source: the source provides radiation in the range in which the absorbing species will absorb or is expected to absorb. A tungsten lamp is used to obtain light in the visible range. In the near ultra violet region a hydrogen lamp, deuterium lamp or xenon lamp may be used. In the infra red region either a Nernst glower which is a hollow rod of yttruin and zirconium oxides heated to about 1450C or the globar which is rod of silicon carbide heated to about 1200 C.

(b) A Monochromator : this allows only one particular wavelength of light to pass through and be incident on the solution. These are either optical filters or diffraction gratings (or both).

(c) An Absorption Cell : in this the solution containing the absorbing species is placed.

(d) A Detector:thismeasuresabsorbance. The detector is made to compare the intensity of light transmitted by a cell containing solvent (I) with that transmitted by a solution containiing the absorbing species (I_0). In the visible and UV regions photoelectric detectors are used. In the infrared region thermal detectors eg bolometers are used.

(e) A Meter calibrated in terms of absorbance and trasmittance.

Absorbance (A) = log I_0/I

Transmittance (T) = I/I_0

Transmittance is given as a percentage (0-100%). The range of absorbance commonly recorded is 0-2.0. The most accurate range for measurement is 0.1 - 0.8 (20 - 85%T).

2. UV-VISIBLE SPECTROSCOPY

2.1 Definition

Interaction of electromagnetic radiation in the range 200-400 nm (UV) and 400-700nm (visible), with matter gives rise to

UV and visible spectroscopy, respectively.

2.2 Principle:

The absorption of light energy by compounds in the visible and UV region involves the promotion of electrons in the σ, π and n molecular orbitals to an antibonding orbital

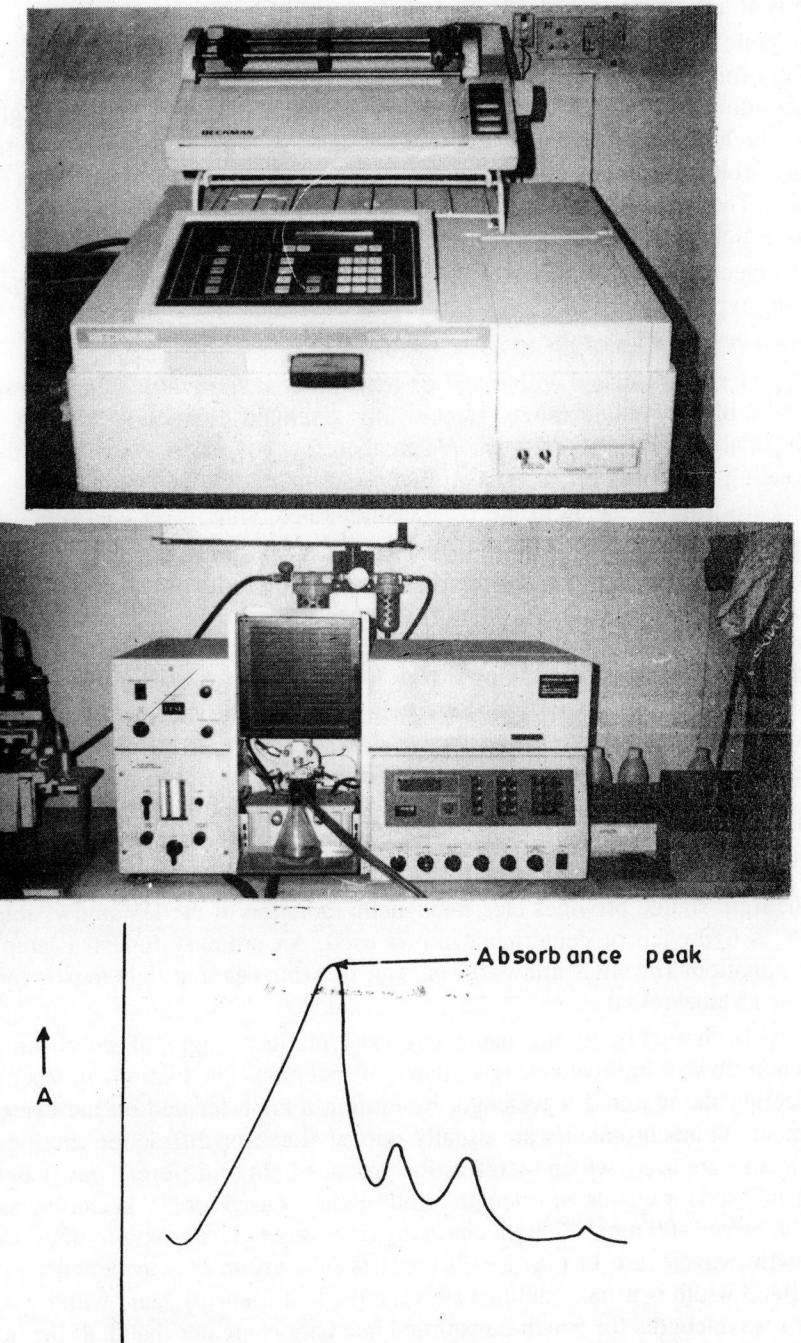

Fig. 3.3 : An arbitrary absorption spectrum showing an absorption peak. (Inset) (a) Scanning UV visible spectrophotometer (a) Atomic absorption spectrometer

which is at a higher energy level.

Organic molecules have several types of molecular orbitals σ and π are called bonding orbitals and are occupied by a pair of electrons in the ground state. There are corresponding σ* (sigma star) and π* (pi star) antibonding orbitals at higher energy levels which are unoccupied in the ground state. A third type of 'n' orbital or non-bonding orbital, also occurs in molecules containing a lone pair of electrons eg oxygen, nitrogen. The electrons here are not directly involved in bonding and are therefore known as non-bonding orbitals.

The electronic transitions ($\rightarrow$) that are involved in the UV and visible regions are of following types in order of energy associated with them (Also see table 1).

$$(\sigma \rightarrow \sigma^*) > (n \rightarrow \sigma^*) > (\pi \rightarrow \pi^*) > (n \rightarrow \pi^*)$$

The energy associated with σ and σ^* transitions is so high that the corresponding λ falls short of the visible range. Hence fully saturated compounds do not show any significant absorption above 200nm and are therefore colourless compounds that contain non-bonding electrons on oxygen nitrogen, sulfur or halogen atoms are capable of showing absorptions owing to n σ^* transitions involving lower energy.

In unsaturated and delocalised systems such as benzene and porphyrins the $\pi \rightarrow \pi^*$ transition is of sufficiently small energy (long λ) to produce an absorption band in the near UV (benzene) or visible (porphyrin) range. This increase in absorbing wavelength due to delocalisation is called a bathochromic shift whereas a decrease in delocalisation caused for example by protonating a ring nitrogen atom causes a hypsochromic shift which leads to decrease in absorbing wavelength. Hyperchromic and hypochromic shifts refer to an increase and decrease respectively in absorbance. Electronic transitions within a molecule may be associated with a given group in the molecule called a chromophore.

2.3 Instrumentation

The spectrophotometer has the following parts (Fig. 3.4)

The light source provides electromagnetic radiation in the UV and visible regions. For UV, a hydrogen or deuterium lamp is used. An ordinary tungsten lamp provides visible radiation. The slit S_1 allows the passage of a thin beam of light to pass through and reach the monochromater.

A monochromator as the name suggests, produces light of only one particular wavelength from a multiwavelength source of radiation. The instrument has a provision for selecting the required wavelength by turning a knob located on the exterior of the instrument. Monochromators are usually optical filters or diffraction gratings or both. Often prisms are used, which by refraction produce light of different wavelengths. Glass prisms are used for visible wavelengths while quartz is used for UV because glass absorbs radiation below 400 nm. The light emerging from any monochromator does not consists of a single wavelength in practice. It consists of a group of wavelengths called band width Band width is usually defined as twice the half intensity band width, which is the range of wavelengths for which transmitted intensity is greater than half the intensity of the chosen wavelength. Band width varies from 5-35 nm depending on the quality of the instrument.

S_2 the slit allows only a thin beam of band width light to pass through. Sample is placed in a cuvette which is optically transparent cell made of glass for visible and quartz for UV light. Commonly used cuvettes have an optical path length of 1 cm. 2.5-3 ml

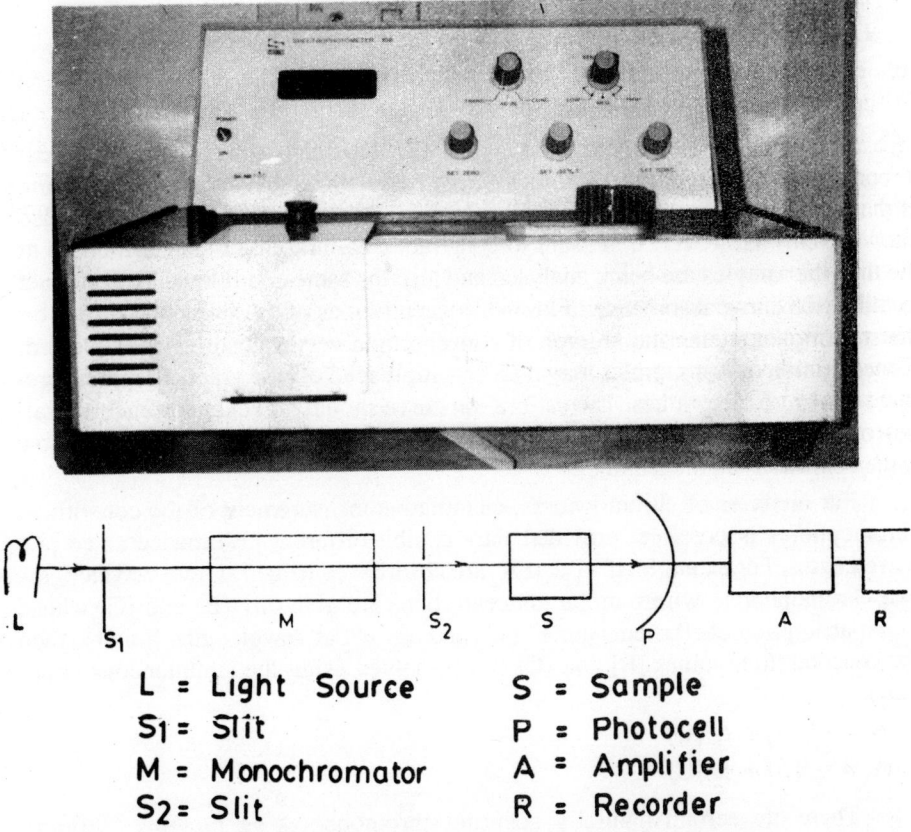

L = Light Source   S = Sample
S_1 = Slit   P = Photocell
M = Monochromator A = Amplifier
S_2 = Slit   R = Recorder

Fig. 3.4 : Parts of a spectrophotometer (inset) a spectropnotometer

sample is required for accurate measurement. There are microcuvettes too, requiring 0.3-0.5 ml sample and are useful when valuable sample and reagents are being used.

The emergent beam from the cuvette reaches the photocell which converts radiation to electrical energy which is amplified detected and recorded. In a photocell, photons impinging on the metal surface in vacuum cause emission of electrons. These are attracted by a positive electrode and hence a current flows which causes a potential difference across a resistor present in the system. This potential difference is recorded on the potentiometer which is calibrated to read absorbance and transmittance. Absorbance is calibrated as log I_o/I while transmittance is calibrated as I/Io where Io and I are intensities of emergent radiation from solution and pure solvent respectively. The corresponding current produced is recorded Photomultiplier tubes are more sensitive than simple photocells. In photomultiplier tubes the emitted electrons are accelerated by high potential and produce secondary electrons by collision with gas molecules present in the tube. This results in large current and so very small changes can be measured.

2.4 Applications

1. Measurement of concentration
2. Growth kinetics
3. Structural studies

4. Enzyme kinetics

5. Effect of pH, ionic strength etc. using difference   spectroscopy

6. Testing purity and homogeneity of sample

7. Identification of compounds.

1. Measurement of Concentration by UV-visible spectroscopy: this is by far the most important application of this technique. From the relationship $A = \varepsilon cl$ provided and at that wavelength for that compound is known   can be calculated since l is also known (1cm). However, it is usual to construct a calibration or standard curve at the time the samples are being analysed and also the same conditions. To construct a calibration curve absorbance of known concentrations of the substance is read on the spectrophotometer and a graph of concentration versus absorbance is plotted. Concentration of test samples may then be simply read off the graph after measurement of absorbance values. The calibration curve should however embrace all values of concentration to be measured and should be measured under exactly the same conditions as the samples.

For mixtures of chromophores, quantitative measurement of the constituent chromophores is possible, provided they exhibit different absorbance at certain wavelengths. For example, if A_1 and A_2 are absorbance values at two wavelengths two chromophores whose molar concentrations are given by [B] and [C] whose molar absorption coefficients are e^B_1, e^B_2 and e^C_1, e^C_2 at wavelengths l_1 and l_2 then the concentration values [B] and [C] can be solved using the simultaneous equations.

$$A_1 = \varepsilon_1^B[B] + \varepsilon_1^C[C]$$
$$A_2 = \varepsilon_2^B[B] + \varepsilon_2^C[C]$$

There are certain naturally occuring chromophores eg proteins (280nm), nucleic acids (260 nm), carotenoides (455 nm) tetrapyrroles (400 nm). However for species which do not absorb in the visible region, a derivative is used. They are made to react quantitatively with some other reagent which after reaction gives a coloured derivative whose concentration is equal to that of the original species e.g. amino acids (280nm) are reacted with ninhydrin to produce a coloured complex whose $l_{max} = 570$ nm. Proteins are treated with Folin Ciocalteau reagent to produce a coloured complex whose $l_{max} = 650$nm. Absorbance at is measured against a reagent blank which contains all reagents but not the substance to be measured. A calibration curve is constructed and concentrations read off it. This technique of producing a coloured derivative is called colorimetry. The only drawback with the technique is that it is destructive. The compound being assayed is destroyed since it is made to form a complex with another compound.

2. Growth Kinetics : in situations where light scattering is the predominant factor causing loss of intensity, measurements of absorbance are actually measurements of turbidity. This reflects number of particles per unit volume. This is useful for constructing growth curves for bacteria.

3. Structural Studies :

(a) Protein structural studies : the spectrum of a chromophore depends on polarity of its environment. If change in polarity of solvent changes spectrum of a constituent amino acid chromophore, without change in conformation of a protein, the amino acid must This is called solvent perturbation. As another example if denaturation exposes a tyrosine present in an internal (hydrophilic) environment to an external (hydrophobic) environment effect of pH, temperature and ionic strength on protein denaturation may be studied.

(b) Nucleic acid structural studies : the absorbance at 260nm of double stranded DNA in solution increases due to denaturation on heating (hyperchromicity).

Hypochromicity on renaturation occurs. Thus effects of pH, temperature, ionic strength on secondary structure of DNA can thus be studied. Solvent perturbation studies can be made for example by replacing normal water by 50% D O in a solution of nucleic acids. D O only changes spectral components due to unpaired nucleotides so fraction of unpaired bases e.g. t-RNA can be estimated.

4. Enzyme kinetics and assays : these are carried out via estimation of change in absorbance per unit time with change in concentration of either substrate or product e.g. binding of a drug (substrate) to a liver microsomal monoxygenase causes a blue shift of cytochrome P 450 component of the enzyme from 420 nm to 390 nm.

5. Difference spectra : these are produced by a double beam spectrphotometer. Here, there are two sample cells, one for reference solution, the other for the sample. Two beams of the same wavelength pass through the sample cells and the difference of absorption by the solutions in the two cells is measured. This enables detection of small changes in absorption.

6. The purity and homogeneity of a compound can be tested : characteristic absorption maxima of different chromophores help in identification of unknown compound in both pure state and in biological preparations e.g. proteins, nucleic acids, chlorophylls. The technique may also be used to detect chemical structures and intermediates occuring in a system by comparing with the spectrum of pure compound under similar conditions. However, for really precise analysis, IR spectroscopy is required.

3. INFRA-RED (VIBRATIONAL) SPECTROSCOPY

3.1 Principle

IR spectra originate from different modes of vibration of a molecule.The absorption of IR energy (10^2 - 10^5 nm) by a compound causes excitation of molecules between vibrational energy levels. Usually from lowest energy vibrational level to the first excited level giving rise to absorption bands refered to as Fundamental bands. Additional (nonfundamental) absorption bands may occur because of the presence of overtones (or harmonics) of reduced intensity, at 1/2,1/3,... the wavelength. (twice, thrice the wave number).

The spectral position is given in terms of wave number or Hertz since it deals with vibrations (wave number = 1/wavelength) When a light wave passes through an atom carrying electrical charge, it is pushed first to one side and then to another. In a molecule having a dipole moment (e.g. H——Cl) the electrical field of a light wave tends to set the charges into oscillation; stretching and compressing the HCl bond alternately. The bond has a natural frequency of vibration depending on the masses of the two atoms and the restoring force of the bond. An incident light waves of the same frequency greatly increases the natural frequency of vibration— resonance is said to occur — and molecules absorb maximum energy at this resonant frequency. This is indicated by an absorpuon peak.

Bond vibration modes are of two types.

(1) Stretching - periodic stretching of bond along bond axis
(2) Bending or deformation type - displacement at right angles to the bond axis (Fig. 3.5).

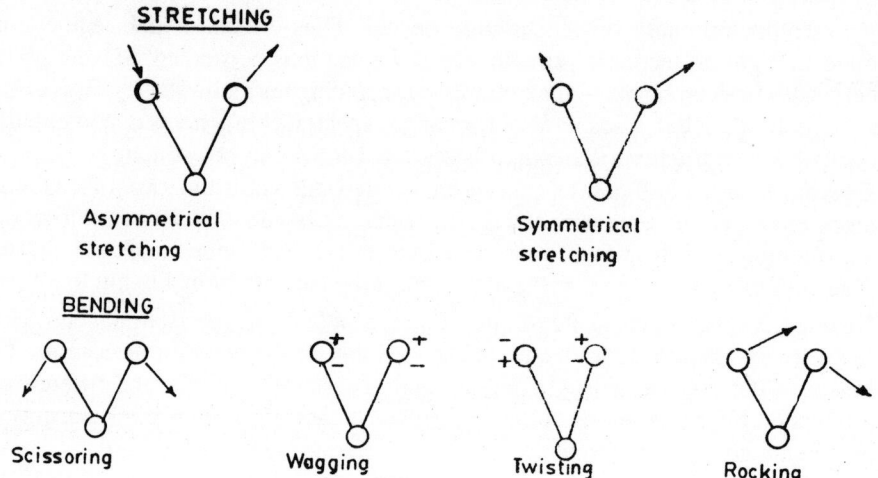

Fig. 3.5 : Bond vibration modes.

Different vibration modes lead to corresponding energy patterns. For a polyatomic molecule there are 3 - 6 modes of vibration of which n - 1 are stretching and 2n - 5 are bending type, n is the total number of atoms in the molecule. Thus C H has 30 fundamental vibrations. However, only those having a transient dipole moment are excited by the radiation. That is to say, that in order for a particular vibration to result in the absorption of IR energy, that vibration must cause a change in the dipole moment of the molecule. Thus IR spectrum of benzene contains less than 30 absorption peaks.

Although IR spectrum is characteristic of a compound the spectra of all molecules contain common characteristics.

(i) In the region 3600-1500 cm absorption due to bonds of the type X—H (e.g. N—H, O—H, C—H)

(ii) Below 1600cm^{-1} - due to C—C, C—N, C—O, C-halogen

(iii) 1300-650 cm^{-1} characteristic of a molecule. This is called the fingerprint region.

3.2 Instrumentation

A common light source for IR radiation is the Nernst glower, as molded rod containing a mixture of zirconium oxide, yttruim oxide and erbium oxide that is heated to around 1500°C by electrical means. Either optical prisms or gratings are used to obtain approximately monochromatic light. The beam is split into two beams one is made to pass through the sample and one through the reference cell. Since glass and quartz absorb IR radiation, metal halides eg NaCl are used as containers of absorbing species. About 1mg substance and 100-200mg of alkali halide are ground together finely and pressed under high pressure to a small disc 1-2 nm in thickness. When equal light intensity is transmitted by both sample and reference beams no signal is produced. Absorbance of sample beam results in inequality of the two transmitting beams folling on the detector which produces a pulsating electrical signal.

The detector is a bolometer or a thermocouple calibrated to give absorbance or transmittance.

3.3 Applications

IR spectrum of a compound is a 'fingerprint' of that compound, hence can be used to identify a pure compound. Correlation charts relate molecular structure to absorption bands. Impurities in a compound may be detected by appearance of extra absorption peaks in the spectrum of a pure compound. IR spectra can distinguish even between isomers of a compound.

Since certain functional groups in a molecule have characteristic natural frequencies that are relatively independent of the molecule. Presence of such functiohal groups can be ascertained in a certain molecule.

Fortunately however, a particular group does not always absorb exactly the same frequency because of environmental influence. Thus it is possible to distinguish between C-H bonds of CH_2 and CH_3.

Since there is a quantitative relationship between absorbance and number of absorbing molecules, quantitative chemical analysis is also possible.

Interfacing IR spectroscopy with Gas Chromatography is a powerful technique for analysing drug metabolites. Its most important application is to study carbondioxide metabolism during photosynthesis and respiration in plants and microorganisms

4. FLAME/ATOMIC ABSORPTION SPECTROSCOPY

4.1 Principle

On absorbing energy of the order of 4×10 KJ mole to 4×10 KJ mole valency shell electrons of atoms get excited to higher energy levels giving rise to absorption line spectra. On returning to the ground state energy given off appears as emission line spectra. Atoms give rise to line spectra and not band spectra like molecules because electronic transitions take place within discrete energy levels characteristic of that atom. Atomic line spectra are therefore said to be fingerprints of atoms and can be used to identify an element quantitative estimations are also possible since the amount of radiation absorbed or emitted is proportional to the concentration of the element.

Flame spectroscopy uses a flame to provide energy for excitation of atoms. The amount of radiation emitted or absorbed is measured as in UV-visible spectroscopy. This is used to quantify the element present in sample which is dissolved in water.

4.2 Instrumentation for Emission Flame Spectroscopy

  (a) Aspirator - which by vacuum action sucks sample solution and takes it to the nebuliser.
  (b) Nebuliser or atomiser produces small droplets of solution which are sprayed into the flame.

(c) Flame serves to volatalise and excite every atom present temperature can be controlled by gas and air pressure controls. This gas used is ually oxy-acytelene flame (2000°C) for higher temperatures of 3500°C a mixture of oxygen and nitrous oxide is used.

(d) Monochromotor- emitted light is made to pass through a monochromator which is adjusted to the characteristic wavelentth which will be emitted by the element.

(e) A Photoelectric Detector as in UV-visible type.

(f) Recorder - the photoelectric detector is connected to a galvanometer calibrated to read concentrations. Alternatively the instrument is calibrated with known concentrations of solution.

The amount of radiation emitted is proportional to the number of atoms excited by the flame. However, not all atoms present are excited hence quantitative measurements are not very precise. The technique of atomic absorption spectroscopy provides more sensitivity and precision.

4.3 Instrumentation for Atomic Absorption Spectroscopy

The element is excited by means of its characteristics spectra produced from a cathode tube whose cathode is made of the element being assayed. The tube contains an inert gas usually Neon at low temperature. A high voltage is used to produce an arc spectrum of the element. Nebuliser, detector and recorder are the same as in emission spectroscopy. In order increase the optical path length of the sample burners producing 10cm flame are used.

In recent years the flame is being replaced by electrothermal heating in a graphite furnace. The sample to be analysed is deposited on a graphite tube in the presence of an inert gas and the temperature raised to 3000°C by electric current. The element in the sample gets volatalised and excited.

4.4 Applications

Since this technique can detect elements as little as less than 1ppm it is widely used in biochemical research for assay of various samples. More than twenty elements can be detected. These include sodium, calcium, potassium iron, manganese, copper, nickel, chromium, zinc, cadmium, lead, lithum and silver.

Diagnosis of certain clinical conditions can be made by observing the departure from usual composition of elements from urine, milk, blood, saliva, and cerebrospinal fluid.

In food chemistry, foodstuffs as also beverages can be analysed for the presence of trace elements or contamination by pesticides when assaying biological samples like cells and tissues ashing is carried out to remove organic molecules.

5. FLUORESCENCE SPECTROSCOPY

5.1 Principle

Fluorescence is a phenomenon whereby a molecule, after absorbing radiation of a particular wavelength, emits radiation of larger wavelength. This is called Stokes shift when the emitted wavelength falls in the visible region, a glow can be seen. Measurement of the intensity of this glow with respect to intensity of incident radiation is called fluorescence spectroscopy or simply fluorimetry.

Absorption and emission are almost instantaneous with a time lag of only seconds approximately during which a molecule exists in excited state. Most organic mlecules in their ground state are singlets (paired) on absorbing radiation they are excited to higher energy state without a change of spin. These are called excited state singlets. Excited state with lowest energy is the first excited singlet. (Fig. 3.6).

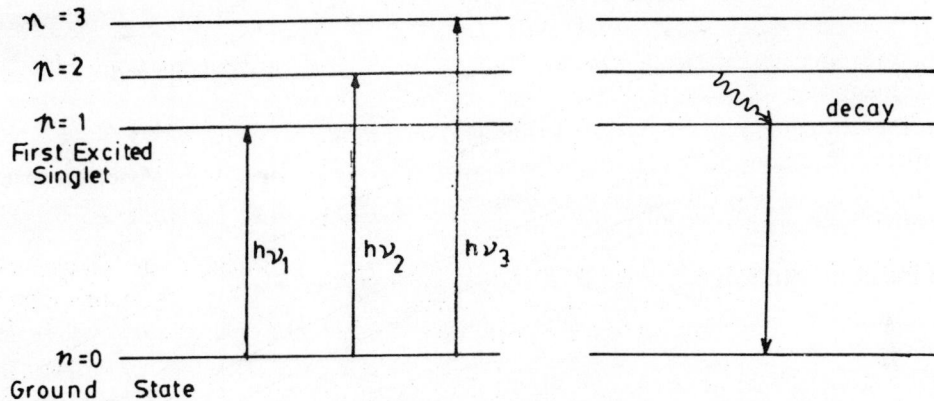

Fig. 3.6 : The Emission process.

Fluorescence occurs when the first excited singlets relax to the ground state. The intensity of fluorescence (I_f) is related to incident radiation (Io) by:

$$I_f = I_o \, 2.3 \, \varepsilon\lambda \, cdQ$$

where,

  c = concentration of fluorescing solution (molar).

  d = light path in the fluorescing solution (cm)

  ε = Molar absorptivity coefficient for the absorbing Material at wavelength λ(dm^{-1} mol^{-1} cm^{-1})

  Q = quantum efficiency which is equal to the number of quanta fluoresced divided by the number of quanta absorbed.

If the initial absorption generates a higher excited state this will relax quickly and non-radiatively to first excited singlet (decay) which may then fluorescence.The non radiative relaxation mechanisms include.

1. Thermal relaxation transfer of energy to molecular and sub-molecular motion e.g. collision, rotation, vibration

2. Photochemical reactions. When such processes win the competition with radiative energy loss, quenching of fluorescence is said to occur.

The efficiency of these non-radiative processes depend on environment of molecule and hence so does fluorescence intensity. Thus fluorescence of an emitter is a probe (indicator) of its enivironment.

5.2 Instrumentation

Fig. 3.7 shows the main components of a spectrofluorimeter. Source is a mercury lamp or xenon arc (M_1) Monochromator is for selecting a chosen wavelength of irradia-

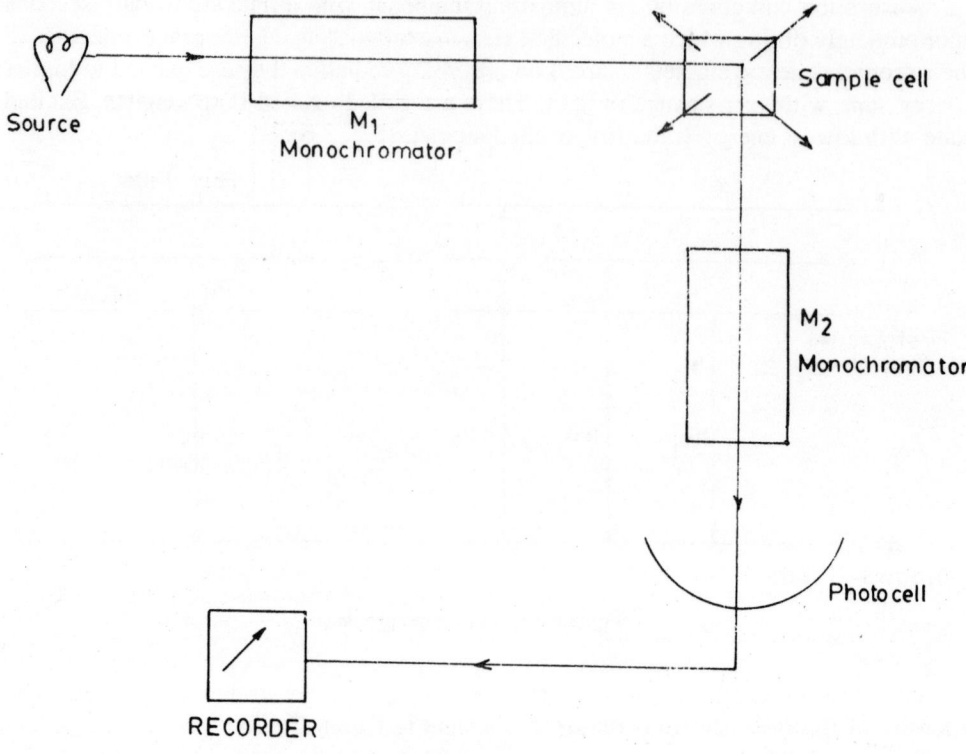

Fig. 3.7 : Main components of a spectrofluorimeter

tion. (M₂) Monochromator enables determination of fluorescence spectrum of a specimen. Photocell detector and recorder as in UV-visible spectrophotometer. The fluorescence from a sample is emitted in all directions but is examined at right angles so that transmitted light does not interfere.

Pre & Post - Filter Effects

Pre -filter absorption reduces the amount of incident radiation reaching fluorescent molecules furthest from the light source and post-filter effects reduces the amount of fluoresscence escaping from the cuvette. Use of a) Microcuvettes (Fig. 3.8a) and/or b) Front Face Illumination (Fig. 3.8b) reduces both pre - and post - filter effects.

5.3 Applications

1. Measurement of concentration : The intensity of fluorescence is directly proportional to concentration of fluorophore (substance emitting fluorescence)according to the relation :

$$I_f = Io \; 2.3 \; c \; l \; Q$$
i.e. $I_f \; \alpha \; c$

hence concentration can be found as in absorption visible spectrophotometry. Since fluorescence has high absolute sensitivity i.e., even very small amounts can be

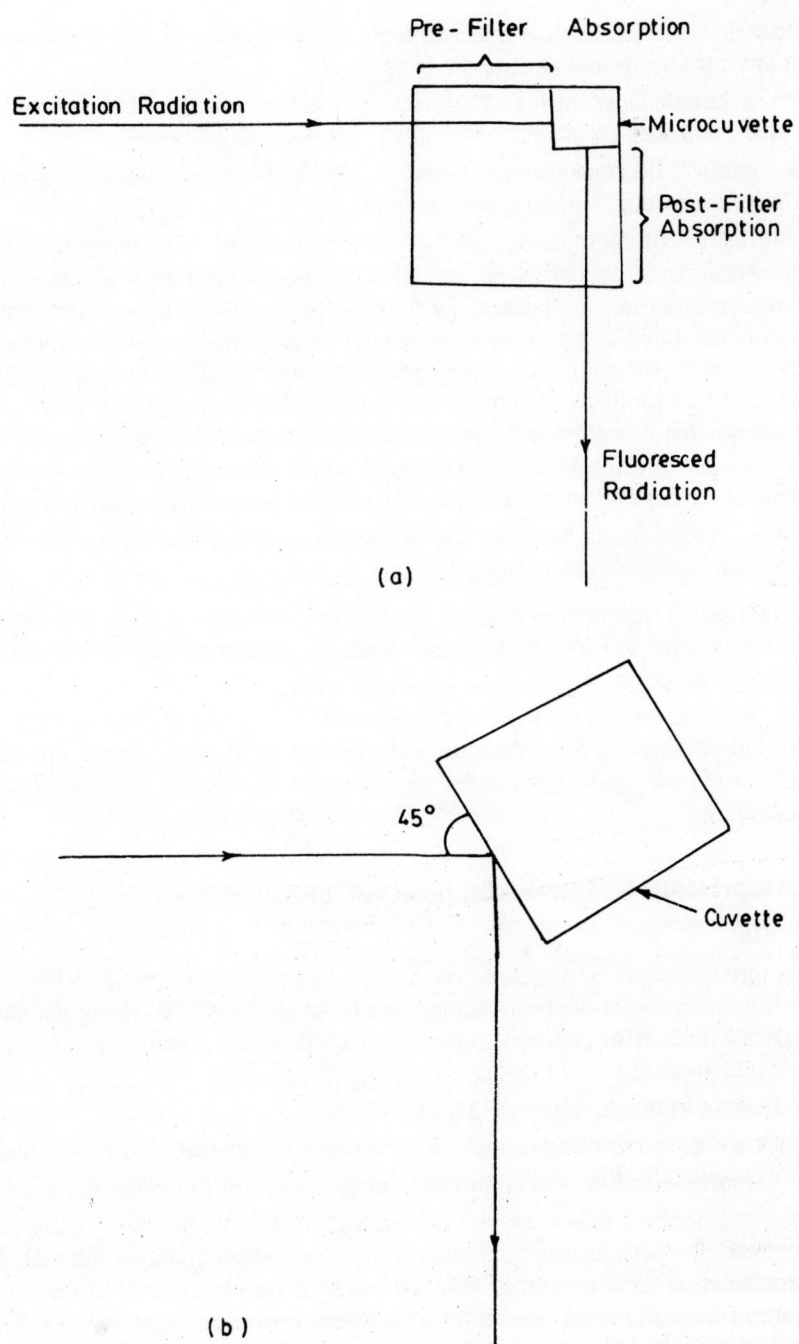

Fig. 3.8 : Reduction of filter effects (a) Using microcuvette (b) Using front face illumination.

detected, it is far better than absorption visible spectrophotometry at concentrations too low for absorption spectral analysis.

If sample lacks intrinsic fluorescence it can be made to bind to a fluorophore or probe and then measure the so called extrinsic fluorescence.

Some extrinsic fluorophores include dansyl chloride, 1-anilinonaphthalene-8-sulphonate (ANS) fluorescein, Ethidium bromide etc.

2. Identification of compounds using excitation spectrum : The comparison of both fluorescence and excitation spectra of a compound may help to identify it. An excitation spectrum is obtained by keeping the emission monochromator of the fluorimeter fixed at a particular wavelength and then successively changing the wavelength of the excitation monochromator and recording the photocell output. The spectrum produced is similar to an absorption spectrum but it has an added advantage that it enables a fluorescencet material to be detected and quantified in the presence of a non-fluorescent material which absorbs at the same wavelength. Hence an absorption spectrum of such a mixture would give overlapping peaks.

3. Kinetic and Structural Studies : Use is made of extrinsic fluorophores to label any biological structure under study.

For example the fluorimetric assay of β-galactosidase enzyme is made using fluorescein di-(-D-galactopyranoside) as substrate. Even a single molecule of enzyme can be detected by this process.

Membrane structure and effects of temperature, pH can be studied using ANS and MNS (N-methyl-2-anilino-6-naphthalein sulphonate) as probes. These contain both hydrophobic and hydrophilic groups and therefore get attached to the water lipid interface of membrane.

6. ELECTRON SPIN RESONANCE (ESR) SPECTROSCOPY

6.1 Principle

ESR is the interaction of an unpaired electron with a microwave field ($\sim 10^{10}$ Hz). As different from other forms of spectroscopy energy levels arise from the application of a static magnetic field. Also only molecules in which there are unpaired electrons can be detected. These include :

   (i) free radicals e.g. $CH_3°$, $C_2H_5°$, $C_6H_5°$,

  (ii) Odd electron molecules such as paramagnetic molecules NO, N_2O and O

 (iii) Paramagnetic ions and complexes such as those of transition metals.

An electron not only moves around the nucleus of an atom but also rotates about its own axis either clockwise or anticlockwise giving rise to spin quantum number, S + 1/2 or -1/2 depending on the direction of spin. This motion may be likened to the flow of an electric current through a loop. Such a flow of current creates a magnetic field. A similar magnetic field is created due to the motion of the electron which therefore has a magnetic moment. This field can interact with an external magnetic field . When an external magnetic field H is applied the electron gets aligned either parellel to it in a low energy state or antiparallel to it in a high energy state depending on the spin of the electron (Fig. 3.9). Thus there are two energy levels after application of magnetic field.

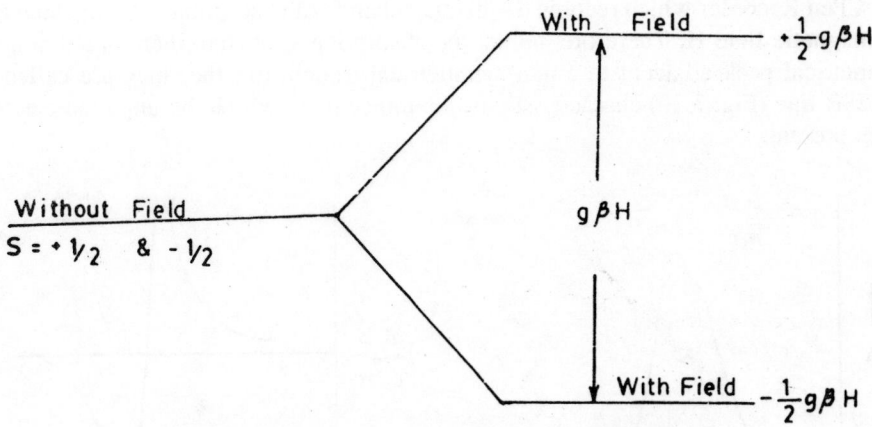

Fig. 3.9 : Energy levels after application of magnetic field.

The unpaired electron can absorb energy from the microwave region of the electro-magnetic spectrum and change from low energy state (spin parellel to H) to high energy state (spin antiparellel to H). This spin reversal (resonance) occurs if energy, E, absorbed is equal to:

$$E = h\nu = g\beta H$$

where, h =Planck's constant

       ν = frequency of wavelength absorbed

       g = a constant called spactroscopic splitting factor

       H = applied magnetic field

       β = magnetic moment of electron called Bohr magneton

From the above relationship it follows that the frequency of absorbed radiation depends on β and H. In practice however, it is usual to keep constant and vary H. This gives rise to an absorption peak when the magnetic field is enough to cause resonance. Such a peak corresponds to a paramagnetic species in the sample. The area under the peak is a measure of the concentration of that species, which may be be quantified if a standard containinng a known amount of unpaired electrons is available. In practice ESR spectra contain many peaks and fine structure due to hyperfine splitting. This is due to interaction of the electron with the magnetic nuclei within the molecule.

6.2 Instrumentation

The requirements of an ESR spectrophotometer are as follows

(a) A Klystron source of monochromatic microwave (3×10^{-2} m/9000 M Hz) radiation.

(b) A Sample cell. Samples must be in the solid state, so biologicalsamples are usually frozen in liquid nitrogen.

(c) A Magnetic Field of 50-500 millitesla surrounding the sample.The magnetic field is generated by electromagnets. Anauxiliary sweep of 10-100 millitesla is also present.

(d) A Detector to determine when the sample absorbs microwave radiation ie the resonance condition. The detector is a bolometer or a crystal detector.

(e) A Pen Recorder which records dA/dH, i.e. change of absorption A, with change of magnetic field H. Therefore, unlike the absorption spectrum, there is a non symmetrical peak adjacent to a non symmetrical trough, together they are called an ESR line (Fig. 3.10) characteristic of the molecule in which the unpaired electron is present.

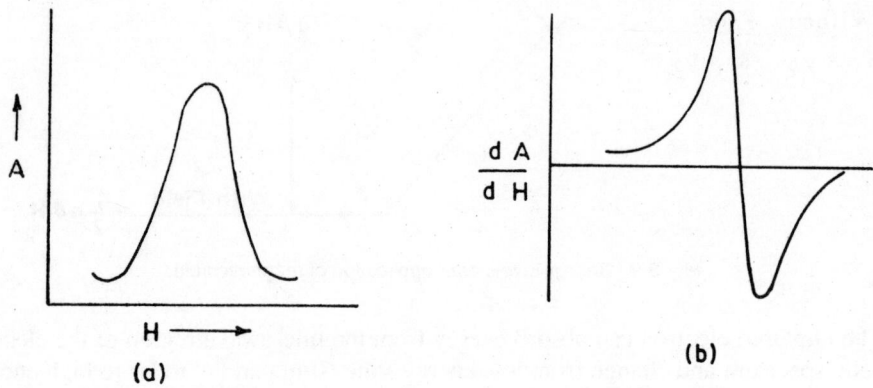

Fig. 3.10 (a) : ESR Absorption curve (b) ESR Line.

6.3 Applications

With the use of synthetic free radicals (spin labels) ESR can now be applied to a wide range of biological systems which lack an endogenous paramagnetic centre. eg. TEMPOL (2,2,6,6-tetramethyl piperidine-1-oxyl) can bind to biological macromolecules which lack unpaired electrons.

Membrane studies : TEMPOL can be bound to glycerophosphatides of membranes and their lateral diffusion can be studied by analysing the ESR signal.

Detection and Identification : ESR signals aid in the recognition of intermediate free radicals occuring in enzymatic reactions, photosynthesis,respiration as also in radiation damaged systems.

Kinetic and Dynamic Studies : For reactions taking less than a nanosecond quantitativeinformation from ESR signals can be used.

7. NUCLEAR MAGNETIC RESONANCE (NMR) SPECTROSCOPY

7.1 Principle

Nuclear Magnetic resonance is the absorption of energy from a radiofrequency ($\sim 10^8$ Hz) of electromagnetic radiation by a system containing unpaired nuclear spins in a strong static magnetic field. The separation of energy levels and hence the frequency of absorption depends on strength of magnetic field.

Like electrons spinning about their own axis, protons in a nucleus also spin either clockwise or anticlockwise about their axis. The spinning positive charge gives rise to a magnetic field with a magnetic moment. Pairs of protons have a net magnetic moment of zero. However, an odd proton in the nucleus imparts a magnetic moment to the molecule, which can interact with an applied magnetic field. In an applied magnetic field

H, it can exist either in a low energy state aligned parellel to the direction of applied magnetic field or antiparellel to it in a high energy state. On absorbing energy from the radiowave region of the electromagnetic region, a proton can change from the low energy state to the high energy state causing resonance to occur and giving rise to Nuclear Magnetic Resonance which is therefore also known as Proton Magnetic Resonance (PMR). For resons already explained NMR can occur only in atoms containing odd number of protons e.g. ^1H, ^{13}C, ^{15}N, ^{19}F, ^3P .

The resonance condition is given by

$\nu = \mu H/hI$

where

ν = frequency of electromagnetic radiation
absorbed

μ = Nuclear magnetic moment

H = Magnetic field strength

h = Planck's constant

I = Nuclear spin quantum number characteristic of an atom.

The above relationship shows that the frequency of radiowaves absorbed during NMR depends on both the atom being studied (described by I) and the strength of the magnetic field. It is common practice, however, to vary the magnetic field, H, and keep frequency constant, in the radiowave region, rather than vice versa case.

7.2 Instrumentation

(a) Source is a radiofrequency transmitter to irradiate the sample

(b) Sample cell containing sample dissolved in a solvent which lacks the atom containing the unpaired electron which is going to be analysed eg in PMR, D_2O or $CDCl_3$ is used.

(c) Electromagnets providing fields of 1-10 tesla, in conjunction with Auxilliary sweep coils to vary the magnetic field over 1-100 millitesla.

(d) Radioreceiver which serves as a detector of the absortpion signal.

(e) Recorder which plots energy absorbed against the magnetic field strength applied.

7.3 Chemical Shifts

Nuclear resonance of a particular atom is not always the same in a given applied static magnetic field. This is because the adjacent electron clouds interact with the applied field to give rise to small induced magnetic fields which alter the effective magnetic field felt by each nucleus. Thus the actual field experienced by a proton depends on its molecular environment e.g. the NMR spectra of ethyl alcohol show that it has three different types of protons; those in the CH_3 group, those in the CH_2 group and that in the OH group. If the induced field opposes the applied field, a higher applief field is required to make the nucleus resonate. Such nuclei are said to be shielded. On the contrary nuclei are deshielded if induced field augments applied field. Such spectral shifts in different structural environments is called Chemical Shifts.

The extent of the Chemical Shift is measured relative to the proton magnetic resonance of tetramethylsilane (TMS) and is called the tau (τ) value.

$$= 10 - \frac{\text{(frequency difference from TMS) x } 10^6}{\text{instrument frequency in Hertz}}$$

The chemical shift is influenced by

(i)   Electronic configuration around nucleus and therefore molecular structure

(ii) Solvent in which sample is dissolved. This is because the process of dissolution involves the bonding electrons of solute and solvent.

(iii) Temperature, in the case of molecules with hydrogen bonding, since temperature affects the strength of the hydrogen bond.

7.4 Applications

NMR spectroscopy is of great importance due to chemical shifts which make the spectra very precise and the ultimate in structural analysis. Chemical shifts are utilised for studying the following situations. Presence of neighbouring aromatic rings can be detected due to abnormal shifts of a particular nucleus. Specific probes can be introduced to cause changes in the shifts makinng it possible to study the effects of the probes on molecular structure.

In a covalent bond the electronic matgnetic moment is zero because electrons are paired. However, the nuclear magnetic moment causes the electrons to be polarised slightly. This effectively transmits the direction of spin of one nucleus to another. Such interaction between like or different spins through the bonding electrons, called spin - spin interactions causes splitting of the NMR absorption peak already separated by chemical shifts. This splitting called hyperfine splitting is used to detect and identify number and kind of chemical groups, bond angles and isomers present. These can be extended to biomolecules e.g. nucleotides, hormones, peptides etc.

Just like other spectroscopic techniques, NMR spectra can be used to determine concentration, measure time course of reactions and probing the environment of molecules (pH, ionic strength proximity to aromatic rings etc.).

7.5. ESR and NMR Compared

Both ESR and NMR provide information about structure of a molecule at the atomic level which is not possible by any other form of spectroscopy. The two differ in the instrumentation involved and practical applications ESR requires a magnetic field of 0.1 to 1 (Tesla while NMR requires a higher (10 fold) field of 1-10 Tesla. ESR absorbs in the microwave region of the spectrum while NMR absorbs in the radiowave region of lesser energy. Although both forms are non-destructive and can be used under near physiological conditions.

NMR is unversally applicable since all biological molecules contain protons and most contain ^{31}P. EPR can only be observed in molecules with unpaiured electrons and this restricts the technique to molecules containing free radicals on paramagnetic centres.

NMR is however, less sensitive than ESR since smaller energy changes are involved. Also, NMR spectra are more complicated due to chemical shifts and spin spin interactions. In contrast, ESR spectra are simpler with only one or two peaks corresponding to paramagnetic centres.

8. CIRCULAR DICHROISM (CD) SPECTROSCOPY

8.1 Principle

CD spectroscopy measures the differential absorption of right (R) and left (L) circularly polarised light as a function of wavelength.

Light consists of electromagnetic waves vibrating in all directions parpendicular to the direction of propagation of light. After passing through a Nicol prism or polaroid light becomes plane polarised i.e., it consists of waves oscillating only in one plane.

When two plane polarised waves of equal amplitude and wavelength but differing in their planes of polarisation by 90 are superimposed, circularly polarised light is obtained. It can be either right (R) circularly polarised or left (L) circularly polarised depending upon the relative positions of the peaks of the two component plane polarised waves.

For an optically active compound $\varepsilon_L \neq \varepsilon_R$ i.e. the molar absorption coefficients of L & R circularly polarised light are unequal. It may absorb either the L or R circularly polarised light more than the other. Maximum absorption occurs when the electric field vector is parellel to the direction in which there is maximum electronic displacement within the absorbing molecules because of the differential absorption of the R and L circularly polarised light, the resultant light is elliptically polarised.

It is this ellipticity (θ) rather than absorbance which is measured as a function of wavelength and a CD spectrum is obtained.

As different from other forms of spectroscopy.

   (i) It requires the use of circularly polarised light as incident radiation.

  (ii) It gives information about the shape or 3-dimensional structure of an optically active molecule.

 (iii) Only optically active molecules can be analysed. This is not a handicap for biological investigations since most biomolecules are optically active eg amino acids (generally of L-configuration, nucleotides (containing the sugars D-ribose and D-deoxyribose) and carbohydrates (D and L configurations) are units from which polypeptides, proteins, nucleic acids and polysaccharides are built up.

8.2 Instrumentation

Fig. 3.11 shows diagramatically the components of a CD spectrophotometer R and L circularly polarised radiation is produced by passing plane polarised light in an electro optic modulator through which an alternating current is passed. Depending on the polarity of the electric field the R or L component of light is transmitted.

The photomultiplier detector produces a voltage proportional to the ellipticity of polarisation of the combined beam falling on it. This is recorded against wavelength by the recorder.

$$\theta = 2.303 \, \Delta E \, \frac{180}{4\pi}$$

where, θ = Ellipticity

ΔE = difference in absorption of R & L waves

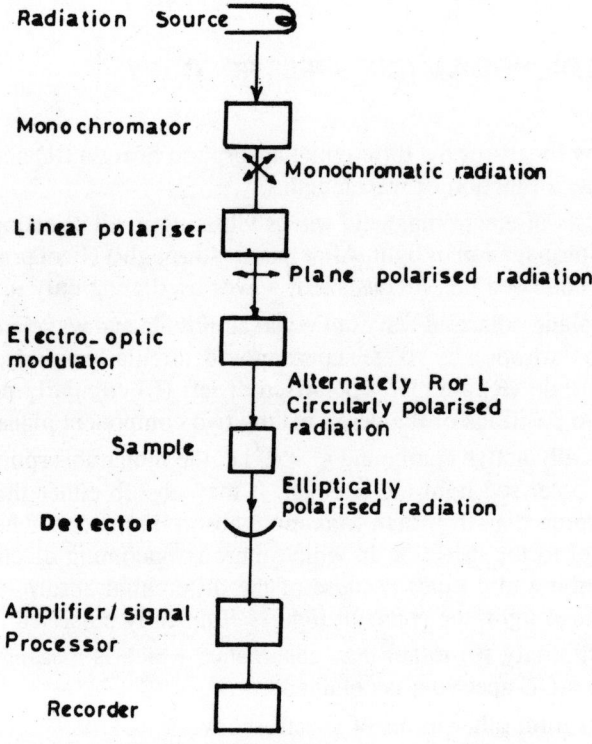

Radiation Source

Monochromator

Monochromatic radiation

Linear polariser

Plane polarised radiation

Electro_optic modulator

Alternately R or L Circularly polarised radiation

Sample

Elliptically polarised radiation

Detector

Amplifier/signal Processor

Recorder

Fig. 3.11 : The main components of a CD spectrometer.

8.3 Applications

Protein conformation : It is possible to study the three-dimensional secondary structure of proteins. The CD spectra of α-Helix, β- conformation and random coil of poly-L-amino acids are known and can be used for calculating the amount of secondary structure present in a protein.

The technique is particularly useful for proteins which cannot be analysed by X-ray diffraction studies.

Nucleic Acid Structure : The CD spectrum of a single stranded nucleic acid can be calculated from its nearest neighbour frequency.

Any difference in the measured CD spectrum can be due to conformational changes in the nucleic acid e.g. double strandedness. These can therefore be studied in detail with the help of a CD spectrum.

4

CENTRIFUGATION

1. PRINCIPLE

Centrifugal means "fleeing a centre". The force acting on a body moving in a circular path can be resolved into two component - normal and tangenital to the path. Centrifugal force (F) is the force on a rotating object which acts tangenitally outwards.

F = m. a.

where,

m = mass of the particle

a = angular acceleration of particle moving in a circle

The angular acceleration is the product of the square of the angular velocity (W) and the radial distance of particle from the axis of rotation i.e.,

$F = M\omega^2 r$

A centrifuge is a device for whirling an object with a high angular velocity. The consequent large acceleration ($\omega^2 r$) is equivalent to increasing the value of g, the acceleration due to gravity and such processes as sedimentation (settling of particles or precipitates out of a solution) can be greatly accelerated in this way. Hence $\omega^2 r$ is expressed as "number times g" or Relative Centrifugal Field (RCF). This is the ratio of the weight of the particle is an applied centrifugal field to the weight of the same particle when acted upon by gravity alone.

In an applied centrifugal field, the rate of sedimentation of a particle suspended in solution depends upon the following factors.

    1. Density and size of particle.

    2. Density and viscosity of medium in which particle is suspended.

    3. Extent to which its shape deviates from spherical.

  1. **Density and size of particle :** The net force on a particle suspended in a medium in a centriffugal field is

$F = M \omega^2 r$

or, $F = \dfrac{4}{3} \pi r_p^3 (\rho p - \rho m) \omega^2 r$ (Since, M = Volume × density) where,

vp = radius of particle
ρp = density of particle
ρm = density of medium
r = radial distance of particle from axis of rotation

2. **Density and viscosity of the medium :** Due to viscosity of the medium, the frictional force fo on a spherical particle, opposes motion through the medium.

$$fo = 6 \pi \eta \, r_p \, v$$

where,

η = coefficient of viscosity
v = velocity of the particle

The particle continues to accelerate till

$$F = fo$$

In this condition,

or, $\quad F = \dfrac{4}{3} \pi r_p^3 (\rho p - \rho m) \omega^2 r \qquad = 6 \pi \eta r_p v$

or, $\quad v = \dfrac{dr}{dt} = \dfrac{2r_p^3}{9\eta} (\rho p - \rho m) \omega^2 r \qquad\qquad$ (1)

or $\quad t = \dfrac{9 \eta}{2r_p^2 (\rho_p - \rho_m) \omega^2 r} = \dfrac{\ln r_b}{r_t}$ $\qquad\qquad$ (2)

where,

r_t = radial distance from axis of rotation to meniscus of liquid medium
r_b = radial distance from axis of rotation to the bottom of the tube.
t = time in seconds

3. **Extent to which its shape deviates from spherical :** The ratio of functional force f on a non. spherical particle to the functional force fo on a spherical particle is equal to one (f/fo=1), while for a non-sperical particle it is greater than one, so that the velocity of sedimentation v is,

or $\quad t = \dfrac{2r_p^2 (\rho_p - \rho_m) \omega^2 r}{9 \eta (f/fo)}$

Thus non-spherical particles sediment at a slower rate.

Thus centrifugation is based on the principle that solution, occurs in an applied centrifuga, field, due to differences in their shapes and masses.

If the composition of the suspending medium is defined, the rate of sedimentation is proportional to $\omega^2 r$ and equation (1) simplifies to $v = s\ \omega^2 r$ where s is sedimentation coefficient. Sedimentation coefficients are usually very small for biological particles, hence a basic unit of 10^{-13} seconds is taken for convenience. This is called the Svedberg unit (S). Thus a sedimentation coefficient of 15×10^{-13} seconds is represented by 15S.

2. Types of Centrifuges

(a) Small bench centrifuges have a maximum rate of 3000-7000g. They are used to precipitate coarse granules, yeast cells etc.

(b) Large capacity refrigerated centrifuges have a maximum rate of 6500g with a capacity of 100 cc. They are refrigerated to control temperature.

(c) High Speed Refrigerated Centrifuges have a maximum rate of 60,000 g, are refrigerated and are used to sediment smaller microorganisms, cellular debris and large cellular organelles.

(d) Continuous flow Centrifuges. Unlike the other centrifuges where tubes are attached to the rotor, here the rotor itself is tubular.

Particles are sedimented against its wall and supernatant continously flows out. Used in large scale harvesting of bacteria.

(e) Preparative Ultracentrifuge has a maximum rate of 600,000 g. The rotor chamber is refrigerated, sealed and evacuated to minimse heat production due to friction between air and spinning rotor.

(f) Analytical Ultracentrifuge has a maximum rate of 500,000g Fig. 4.1. In addition to the parts of a preparative ultracentrifuge monitoring of sedimenting material is achieved by utilising ultra-violet absorption system observing differences in refractive index using

  (i) Schlieren optical system or

  (ii) Rayleigh interferometric system

In the Schlieren optical system, when light passes through different density zones, it is refracted at the boundary between these zones. In the sedimenting material in the analytical cell, a boundary is formed between the solvent which has been cleared of particles and remainder of the solution containing the sedimenting material. Light is refracted at the boundary. Schlieren system plots refractive index gradient against distance along the analytical cell. Concentration can be determined from area of the peak.

3. TYPES OF CENTRIFUGATION

  3.1 Differential Centrifugation

  3.2 Density Gradient Centrifugation

3.1 Differential Centrifugation

This is based on differences in sedimentation rate due to differences in size and density of particles. Particles of greater density sediment faster during a given period of applied centrifugal field. The material to be sedimented is divided into a number of fractions by step-wise increasing the applied centrifugal field. Material sediments to give a pellet while the supernatant has unsedimented material. The supernatant is then sedimented at a higher speed to pellet smaller molecules.

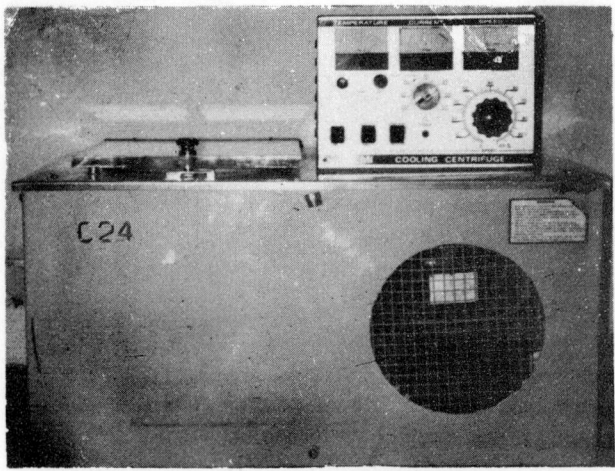

(a) Cooling centrifuge

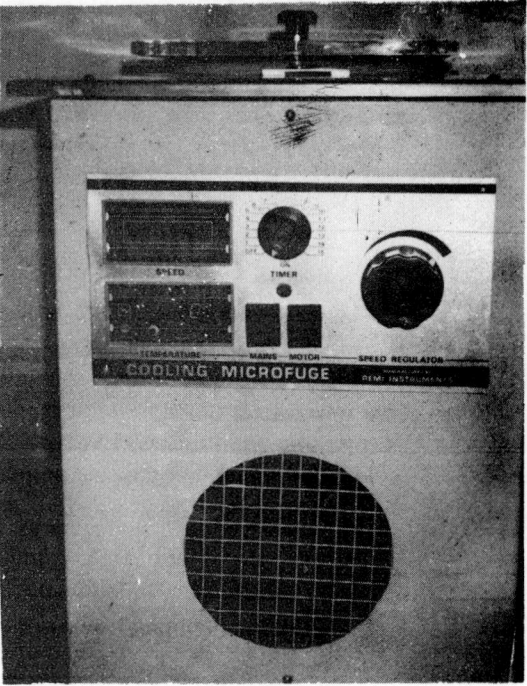

(b) Cooling microfuge

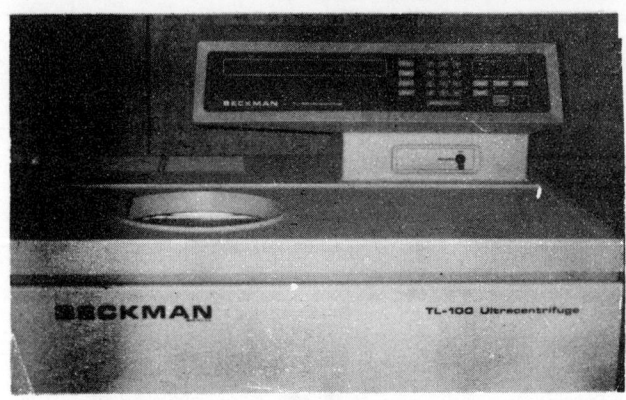

(c) Analytical ultracentrifuge.

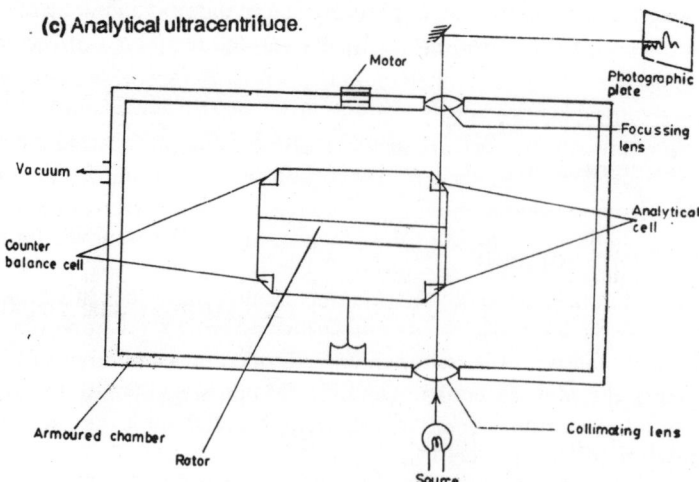

Fig. 4.1 : The Analytical ultracentrifuge insects

3.2 Density Gradient Centrifugation

In this, the density of the medium increases towards the bottom of the tube.

3.2.1 Density gradients can be prepared by

(a) Discontinuous technique : solutions of decreasing density are carefully layered over each other using a pipette.

(b) Continuous technique : requires the use of a gradient former. This consists of two precision bored cylindrical chambers of identical diameter interconnected at the base by a tube containing a control valve which regulates mixing.

(c) Self forming density gradients : concentrated solution of liquid is centrifuged. The opposing forces of centrifugation and diffusion result in the formation of a gradient.

In the Rate Zonal method of density gradient centrifugation, the sample is layered on top of a pre -formed density gradient (Fig. 4.2), whose maximum density is never more than the densest particle in the sample.

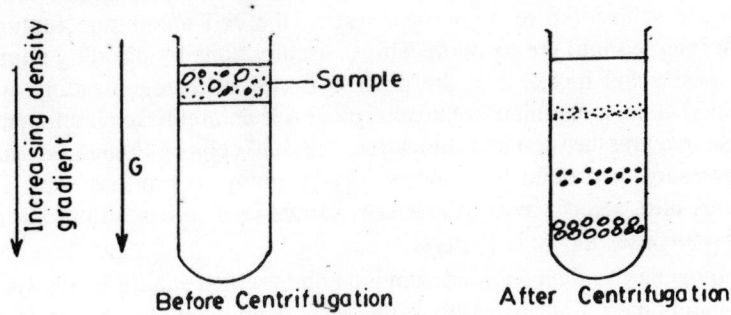

Fig. 4.2 : Rate Zonal centrifugation.

In an applied centrifugal field particles separate according to their relative velocities, in a given period of time, and form distinct zones. Usually centrifugation is stopped before equilibrium position is reached, therefore, pelleting does not occur.

In the Isopycnic method, a pre -formed density gradient is not required. Centrifugation of the medium and sample together allow formation of a self forming density gradient simultaneously with redistribution of particles and subsequent banding at isopycnic positions. The maximum density of the gradient formed is always greater than the density of the densest particle. In a centrifugal field sedimentation occurs until buoyant density of particle is equal to density of medium. Particles therefore float on a buoyant cushion of denser medium at this equilibrium position. Pellet is never formed even if centrifugation continues over a long period.

A hole is then punched at the bottom of the centrifuge tube and fractions are collected and analysed .

4. APPLICATIONS

4.1 Cell Fractionation and Metabolic Studies

The metabolic function of individual cell organelles and soluble components within the

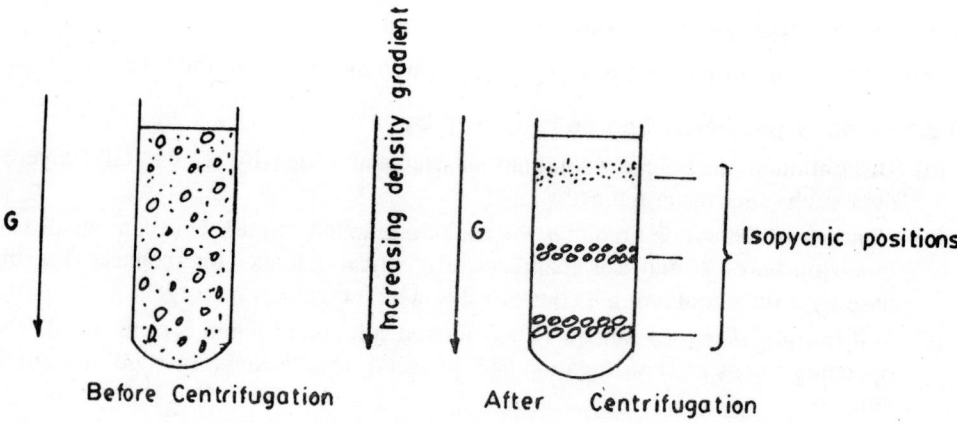

Fig. 4.3 : Isopycnic centrifugation

cell can be studied by separating the cell components from each other by centrifugation. When cells are subjecdted to high shear forces, the cell membrane ruptures and the contents are released into the medium. This is usually done by grinding animal or plant tissue in a pestle and mortar and the process is called hemogenisation. Chloroplast material, blood cells, unicellular organisms, plant and animal tissue homogenates can be ruptured also in a pressure cell and sonication. Pressure cells eg French Pressure Cell use hydraulic pressure controlled by a motor -driven pump to produce shear forces. The sonicator uses ultra-sonic waves to produce cavitational forces within the suspending medium which causes the cells to burst.

The homogenate is then suspended in a medium which should be cheap, uncharged and metabolically inert. Following this, either density gradient centrifugation or differential centrifugation can be used to separate the cell components. As already described in density gradient centrifugation the cell components band at the isodensity positions. In differential centrifugation the homogenate is separated into a number of fractions by centrifuging at various g values. The cell components sediment to form a pellet at different rates according to their size and density. For example rat liver homogenate can be separated into different components by subjecting to differential centrifugation.

Centrifugation conditions g values	time (min.)	Major components in fraction
500	5	Nuclei, whole cells
8000	10	Mitochondria, some lysosomes
15000	10	Mitochondria, lysosomes
100,000	60	Microsomes (membrane fragments, largely ER) ribosomes.
Final supernatant		Soluble components of the cell.

Liver homogenate (20 % in ice cold 0.25 mol/l sucrose)

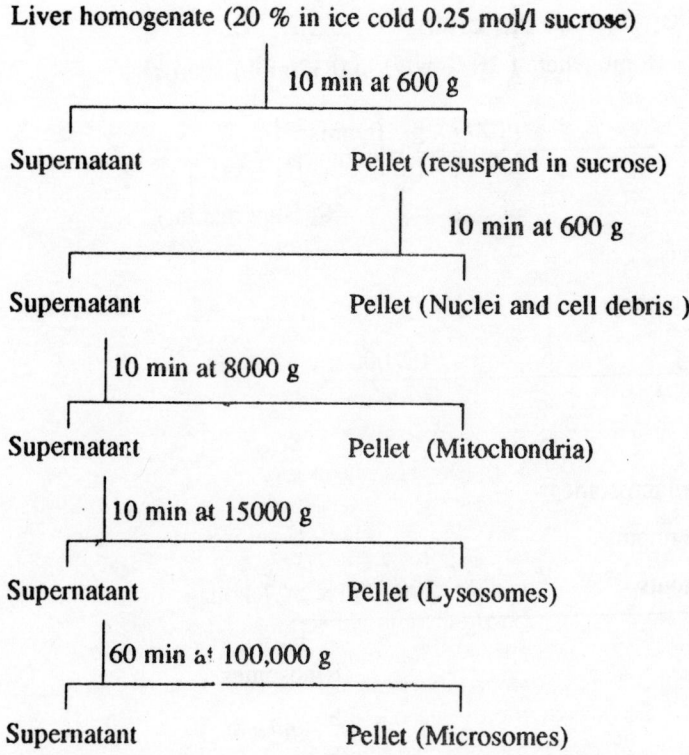

Certain tissues eg. pig brain tissues are very heterogenous in nature so that differential centrifugation gives rise to fraction of a different composition to those from ret liver. Each fraction contains a very complex mixture of components and density gradient centrifugation is required to purify them further. This is illustrated in the following flow chart.

Differential centrifugation of pig brain

Homogenate (10 % w/v) in 0.32 mol/l sucrose

1000 x g, 10 mins.

P$_1$ (Pellet)   S$_1$ (supernatant)

Nuclei, Cell debris

Large myelin fragments

10, 000 x g , 20 min

P$_2$ S$_2$

Mitochondria, Synaptosomes

Small Myelin fragments

Membrane fragments   100, 000 x g , 1 hour

P$_3$ Ribosomes

Microsomes   Cytoplasm

Densty gradient centrifugation of pellet P

Suspended in 2 % w/v ficoll in 0.25 mol/l sucrose

Increasing
density gradient
of ficoll in   Membrane
sucrose   Synaptosomes   Diluted with 0.25
                       Mitochondria   mol/l sucrose

57 500 x g, 45 min.   72, 500 x g, 20 min Pellet

re suspended in ice cold
water

Increasing   Membrane sheet, Synaptic vesicles
density   Synaptosomal membrane
gradient of   Synaptosomes, Mitochondria
sucrose   Mitochondria

A hole is punched in the bottom of this centrifuge tube usually made of plastic. Alternatively the tube is frozen solid and cut into slices for analysis.

4.2 Molecular Weight Determination

Molecular weights of the biological materials can be determined using the Analytical Centrifuge. The molecular weight, M, is related to the sedimentation coefficient s, of a molecule by the following equation

$$M = \frac{RTs}{D(1 - v\rho)}$$

where,

D = Diffusion coefficient of the molecule.

* = partial specific volume of the molecule (volume increase when 1g of solute is added to an infinite volume of solution)

ρ = density of solvent at 20°C.

The sample containing the molecule is centrifuged at high speeds in an ultracentrifuge. The molecules move radially outward thereby creating a distinct boundary between the solvent containing the molecules and the solvent without it. This boundary moves radially outward depending on the sedimentation coefficient of the molecule. The movement is recorded by either the Schlieren or Rayleigh optical system, thereby D is found

since $v = s\omega^2 r$

$$s = \frac{v}{\omega^2 r}$$

ω^2, r and v are known hence s can be found and used to calculate M.

As a better alternative, equilibrium sedimentation can be used to determine the molecular weight. Centrifugation is continued till the solute particles acquire a static position in the tube. This happens when there is an equilibrium between sedimentation due to centrifugal and field and movement of particles in opposite direction due to diffusion. Using the concentration gradient, the molecular weight can be calculated from the formula.

$$M = \frac{2RT \ln (C_2/C_1)}{\omega^2(1 - ve) (r_2^2 - r_1^2)}$$

where C2 and C1 are concentrations of solute at distances r2 and r1 from the axis of rotation.

4.3 Detection of Concentrational Changes

Since the rate of sedimentation varies with not only the size but also the shape of the molecule, changes in conformation eg change of ds DNA to ss DNA causes it to band at different isodensity positions thereby revealing the change in conformations.

5

MANOMETRY

1. INTRODUCTION

Manometry is a technique for measuring pressure of gases and vapours. It has been successfully employed in biological studies to measure uptake and evolution of gases, usually O_2 and CO_2 in living systems. The pressure changes are used to quantify, that is, measure the amount of gases being absorbed or taken up. These studies are particularly useful for study of intermediate steps of metabolism. The beginning and end of some major metabolic pathways have been identified from balance - sheet studies of metabolic input and output of intact organisms. In this way, ethanol and CO_2 were found to be end products of glucose fermentation in yeast. To identify whether or not a particular pathway is operating, inference is made from the yield of microorganisms growing on a particular substrate or by measuring gaseous exchange which requires preliminary knowledge of stoichiometry and pathways of dissimilation.

2. PROCEDURE

Manometric studies are carried out in a small flask attached to a manometer which measures changes in the amount of gas in the flask. The flask is always immersed in a water bath of controlled temperature and is constantly shaken to ensure efficient gas exchange Fig. 5.1 shows a constant volume Warburg Manometer. It consists of a Warburg flask attached to the inner arm of a manometer which is fitted with a three-way stopcock. The Warburg flask consists of a main vessel with a central well. Attached to the main vessel is a side arm which is equipped with a gas vent. The flask may be opened to the air by twisting the gas vent so that the hole is lined up with the slot in the ground glass joint of the side arm. In operation the three-way stop cock and the gas vent are turned so that the system is selaed.

Before reading the fluid reservoir thumbscrew is adjusted so that the fluid level in the inner arm of the Manometer (the closed end) comes to a fixed position usually 150 mm on the scale. Thus the volume of the system remains constant during all observations.

Gas evolution or uptake is measured by changes in the height of the column of the fluid in the outer arm of the Manometer.

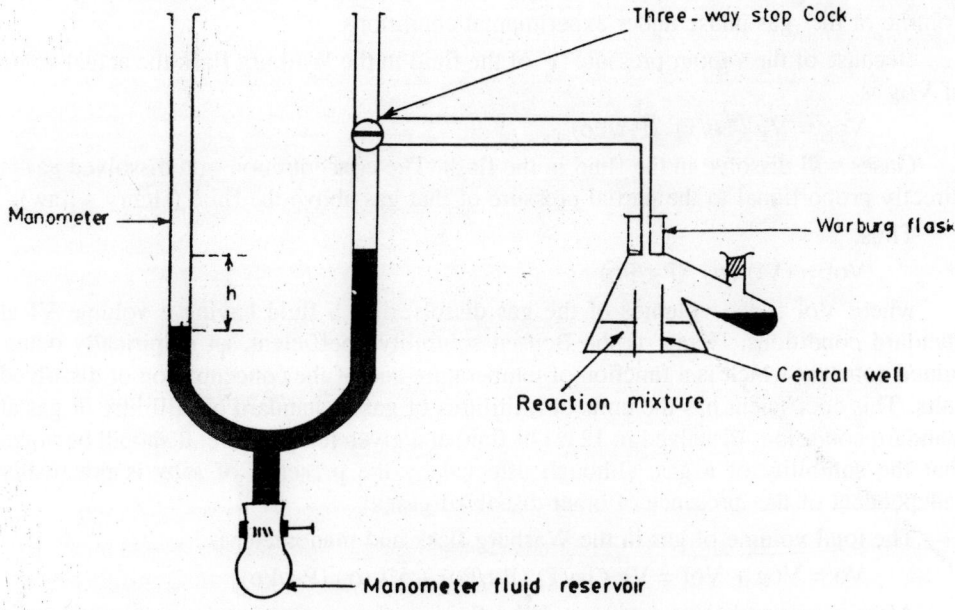

Fig. 5.1 : A constant volume warburg manometer.

In Fig. 5.1, CO_2 is being absorbed in the experimental flask and the resulting decrease in pressure forces the fluid level in the inner arm to rise and in the outer arm to fall. At regular intervals the meniscus of the fluid in the outer arm is returned to the reference point P by withdrawing fluid into the reservoir using the adjustable clamp. The volume of gas exchanged,

Q, is obtained by multiplying the change in the height of the fluid column in the outer arm by a factor known as the flask constant, Or K by the relation:

Q = hK

This factor relating gas exchange and change in the outer arm of a constant volume manometer is a function of the density of the manometer fluid, the temperature the particular gas exchange and the volume of the gas and liquid phases.

2.1 Derivation of the Flask Constant

From Boyle's law, we get the relation

PV = RT

where P is the gas pressure in millimeters of manometer fluid, V is the volume of gas, R is the gas constant and T is the absolute temperature in °K.

we have,

PV/T = R

PV/T = PoVo/To

where the subscript zero refers to standard conditions i.e. a pressure of one atmosphere (760 mm Hg) and temperature of 270° K. We can then write

Vog = Vg (To/T) (P/Po)

where Vog is the volume of the gas phase at standard conditions and Vg is the volume of the gas phase under experimental conditions.

Because of the vapour pressure 'r' of the fluid in the Warburg flask the actual value of Vog is

$$Vog = Vg \ (To/T) \ (P-r/Po)$$

Gases will dissolve in the fluid in the flask. The concentration of a dissolved gas is directly proportional to the partial pressure of that gas above the fluid (Henry's Law).

Thus,

$$Vof = (Vf) \ (\alpha) \ (P-r/Po)$$

where Vof is the volumes of the gas dissolved in a fluid having a volume Vf at standard conditions. Here   is the Bensen solubility coefficient, an empirically determined constant which is a function of temperature and of the concentration of dissolved salts. This coefficient has the units of millilitres of gas at standard of millilitre of gas at standard conditions dissolved in 12 ml of fluid at a given temperature. It shoudl be noted that the solubility of a gas, although affected by the presence of salts is practically independent of the presence of other dissolved gases.

The total volume of gas in the Warburg flask and manometer is

$$Vo = Vog + Vof = Vg \ (To/T) \ (P-r/Po) + Vf \ (\alpha) \ (P-r/Po)$$

After a gas exchange occurs and the fluid in the inner arm of the manometer is readjusted to the original reference point (for example 150 ml) the height of the fluid in the outer arm of the manometer will change by 'h' mm and the pressure in the closed system will be (P-r)-h (written as gas uptake). The total volume of gas at the conclusion of the gas exchange will be

$$Vo = Vg \ (To/T) \ ((P-r)-h/Po)   + Vf( ) \ ((P-r)-h/Po)$$

Accordingly the volume of gas exchanged, Q, is equal to the differences between Vo and V'o.

$$Q = Vo - Vo'$$
$$Q = (Vg \ (To/T) \ (P-r/Po) + Vf \ (\alpha) \ (P-r)/Po)$$
$$-(Vg \ (To/T) \ ((P-r)-h/Po) + Vf(\alpha)(P-r)-h/Po)$$
$$Q = (Vg/Po) \ (To/T) \ (h) + (Vf/Po) \ (\alpha) \ (h)$$
$$Q = h \ (Vg \ (To/T) + Vf \ (\alpha)/Po)$$
$$Q = hK$$

The quantity K is the flask constant. The term h is expressed as mm of manometer fluid. The temperature To and T are 273°K and 273°K + t°C respectively. The volumes Vg and Vf are expressed as microlitres and Po is expressed as mm of manometer fluid. Since the manometer fluid (Kreb's formulation) has a density of 1.033g/ml and the density of Hg is 13.6 g/ml.

$$Po = 760 \times 13.6/1.033 = 10,000 \ mm.$$

The constant K is expressed in terms of microlitres of gas per millilitres fluid. The value of Q is ths the volume change of gas at standard conditions and has the dimension of microlitres μll). This means that Q devided by 22.4 is equivalent to the number of micromoles of gas exchanged.

2.2 Evaluation of the flask constant (K)

The flask constant K can be determined by an evaluation of Vg, the volume of the gas phase, since the other terms are known.

See Table 5.1 for values of (Bensen solubility coefficients) for O , CO and N solubility of gases in water.

Table 5.1

Temperature °C	O_2	CO_2	N_2
20	0.0310	0.878	0.0152
25	0.0283	0.759	0.0143
30	0.0261	0.665	0.0134
35	0.0244	0.592	0.0126
37	0.0239	0.567	0.0123
40	0.0231	0.530	0.0118

The volume of the gas phase is the difference between the total volume of the system (including the volume of the portion above 150 mm in the inner arm of the manometer) and the volume of the fluid in the flask, Vf.

The most accurate method of determining the total volume is to weigh the amount of mercury required to fill the system, but this is tedious and time consuming. A simpler method is to find h (the change in mm of fluid in the outer arm) when a known amount of gas (Q) is exchanged. Since h and Q are known, as are T, α, Vf then Vg, the total volume of flask can be calculated. For example the oxidation of hydrazine by ferricyanide is used to determine Vg and hence K.

$$N_2H_4 + 4Fe(CN)_6^{-3} \longrightarrow N_2 + 4Fe(CN)_6^{-4} + 4H^+$$

Since this is a quantitative conversion the quantity of nitrogen evolved (Q) in the presence of excess hydrazine is calculated from the amount of ferricyanide added to the reaction mixture. The experimental procedure is as follows:

Materials required:
1. Warburg Constant Temperature Bath and shakes, Manometer and Warburg Flasks
2. Potassium ferricyanide reagent. This is freshly prepared 823 mg ferricyanide is dissolved in 100 ml of glass distilled water and is stored in a brown bottle with a loosely fitting glass stopper.
3. Hydrazine reagent. 1.0 gm hydrazine sulfate is dissolved in 70 ml water. 30 ml 1N NaOH is added.
4. Kreb's manometer fluid. 4.4g anhydrous NaBr, 30 ml Triton - X - 100 and 30 mg Evan's blue in 100 ml water.
5. Anhydrous lanolin
6. Chloroform
7. Pipe cleaners
8. Stopcock grease and pipe cleaners

Place 2 ml ferricyanide reagent and 0.6 ml water in the main vessel (not the center well) of a Warburg flask. Place 0.5 ml of hydrazine reagent in the side arm. After removing old grease with chloroform, apply sufficient lanolin to the sides of the glass joint of the Manometer to ensure tight seal. Seal the joint of the flask to the manometer with a rotary motion. Be sure that lanolin is evenly distributed on the joint with no lines or streaks. Then secure the flask to the manometer with a rubber band or steel spring. Grease the gas vent joint with lanolin, insert and seal by rotating to the appropriate position to close the system from the atmosphere. Apply stopcock, grease, not lanolin to the threeway stopcock. Turn the stopcock so that the system is open to the air and place the assembled respirometer in the constant temperature bath in such a way as to avoid mixing the two reagents in the Warburg's flask. Prepare a control flask, termed a thermobarometer by placing 3.1 ml water in a Warburg flask of similar size and attaching the flask to a manometer. Place the thermobarometer beside the first respirometer. Allow the respirometer and thermobarometer to equilibrate in the constant temperature bath while shaking them for 5 min with the stopcocks open.

Seal the respirometer but not the thermobarometer by turning the stopcock. Adjust the level of the manometer fluid so that the fluid level in the outer arm is near the lowest mark on the scale and the fluid level in the inner arm is at 150 mm.

Make the initial reading of the respirometer. Since all readings are constant volume readings all readings of the fluid level of the outer arm must be preceded by an adjustment of the inner arm to some fixed point in this case 150 mm. Continue to note and record the manometer reading at 2 minutes intervals until the fluid level of the outer arm remains essentially constant. Then adjust the inner arm of the thermobarometer to 150 mm, close the stopcock and record the fluid level of the outer arm of the thermobarometer. Both the respirometer and the thermobarometer are now temperature equilibrated.

After equilibration, tip the contents of the side arm of the calibration flask into the main vessel in the folowing manner. First place the index finger firmly over the tip of the outer arm of the manometer. Then quickly withdraw the respirometer from the water bath in an upright direction and, still covering the tip of the outer arm, tilt the flask so that the contents of the side arm run into the main vessel. Then tilt the flask in the reverse direction, allowing the contents of the main vessel to flow into the side arm. Quickly repeat emptying the side arm into the main vesel allowing the entire contents to drain into the main vessel, and return the respirometer to the constant temperature bath. This entire operation should be performed quickly.

After shaking the flask for 2 minutes in the bath, take readings of both the thermobarometer and respirometer after adjusting the fluid level to 150 mm as before. Repeat readings at 2 minutes until the reaction is complete, as indicated by the cessation of gas evolution.

Note that according to the reaction

$$N_2 H_4 + 4 Fe (CN)_6^{-3} \longrightarrow N_2 + 4 Fe(CN)_6^{-4} + 4 H$$

4 moles of ferricyanide liberate 1 mole (22.4 l) of N_2.

4 μ moles of ferricyanide liberate 1 μ mole N_2. Since the molecular weight of ferricyanide is 329.3g, therefore 4 x 329.3 μg liberate 22.4 μl N. We took 2 ml of

ferricyanide solution containing 8.23 g/l ferricyanide. So in 2 ml there are 16.46 mg (8.23x2/1000). Therefore 16.46 mg liberate = $16.46 \times 22.4/1.317 = 280 \mu l$ N_2.

Using this known volume of gas evolved (calculated as shown above from the known quantity of K_3 Fe $(CN)_6$ in the flask), Vf, α from Table 5.1, the temperature and the change in the volume of fluid in the outer arm in millimeters (h) , Calculate the volume of gas (Vg) in the system from the equation.

$$Q = h (Vg (To/T) + Vf (\alpha)/Po)$$

Now using this value of Vg, the α values of table 5.1 and fluid volume of 3.1 ml, calculate values for flask constant, K, at the temperature of the bath for O_2 and CO_2. Record these values for future experiments.

2.3 Removing Bubbles from Manometer Column

If the column of fluid is broken in the manometer it may be readily joined again by rapidly compressing the rubber reservoir with the finger and then releasing the pressure slowly.

Repeating this soon raises the bubbles to the surface of the liquid.

2.4 Adding Manometric Fluid

Draw the fluid into a hypodermic syringe. Jab the inside through the rubber tubing near the base of the reservoir and inject the desired quantity of fluid. The rubber tubing reservoir may be filled before it is attached to the Manometer and addition of fluid can be made through the open arm of the manometer.

2.5 Reading the Manometer after it has passed the Graduated Range

If gas release or uptake is more rapid than anticipated, the fluid end in the open arm of a Warburg manometer may come to rest below or above the graduated range when the fluid in the closed arm of the manometer is adjusted to its reference point. The method follows. Adjust the fluid in the closed arm until the in the open arm is on the scale. The distace one has moved the fluid in the closed arm from the zero point is called 'e' . Record the reading in the open arm. Adjust the closed arm so that the fluid is a distance '2e' from the zero point. Record the reading in the open arm. The difference between the two readings of the open arm is the amount to be added or substracted from the first reading to give the actual reading if the closed arm had been at the zero point.

2.6 Reference Points

The reference point should be chosen to make maximum use of the graduated scale of the Manometer. When gas uptake are measured 250 mm is a convenient point, when gas evolution is measured 50 mm is convenient. 250 mm also may be used as a reference point for gas release if one attaches a length of rubber tubing to the open arm of the Manometer and gently blows the manometer fluid to the level of about 50mm in the open arm and 250mm in the closed arm before closing the stopcock.

The following method using 150 mm as the reference point is suggested by P.P. Cohen. In measuring gas uptake the manometer fluid is set with the stopcock open near the bottom of the scale. In measuring gas release the opposite type of setting is employed. This permits the use of one reference point for both uptake and release of gas and makes maximum use of the graduated scale.

3. APPLICATIONS

Warburg measurements are of great value in metabolic study of many reactions which involve gas exchanges. For example glycolysis can be assayed by measuring CO_2 evolution whereas aerobic respiration of mitochondria is assayed by measuring O_2 uptake Decarboxylations are assayed by measuring the amount of CO_2 evolved and organic acid production can be measured as CO_2 released from a bicarbonate buffer. When studying these reactions it is best to use the maximum possible scale, on the outer manometer arm in order to allow greater latitude in enzyme and substrate concentration. Enzyme studies directly or indirectly involve production or utilisation of gases, hence manometric methods have been used extensively in assaying enzyme activity. The features of the manometric techniques used for enzyme study are:

1. The need for only small amounts of enzyme preparation.
2. The accuracy and speed of estimation and
3. The speed with which one can study the effects of inhibitors substrate concentration, pH and other aspects of kinetics.

Since uptake of O_2 and evolution of CO_2 can be studied simultaneously, the respiratory Quotient (RQ) can be determined using the relationship.

$$R\,Q = \frac{CO_2 \text{ evolved}}{O_2 \text{ absorbed}}$$

This can give information about the nature of the substrate since carbohydrates have an RQ of 1, proteins of approximately 0.8 and fats of approximately 0.7. Also, the efficiency, with which a particular substrate is being utilised can be studied.

6

ELECTROPHORESIS

1. PRINCIPLE

The principle of electrophoresis is very simple i.e. a charged ion or group will migrate towards one of the electrodes when placed in an electric field.The velocity v in centimeter per second of the charged ion is the product of the ion's net electrophoretic mobility μ, in cm^2/volts and strength of the field E also known as potential drop in volt /cm.

$$v = \mu E$$

The net electrophoretic mobility is a physical constant under defined electrophoretic conditions.

$$\mu = v / E = q / 6\pi \ \eta$$

Thus μ depends upon the viscosity of the medium η,size and shape of the molecule as defined by r ,the radius of the molecule and charge q on the molecule. Thus molecules are separated on the basis of differences in charge to mass ratio.The size and magnitude of charge carried by the ion or groups varies according to the ionic strength and pH of the medium in a characteristic manner. Separation of molecules can therefore be achieved by selecting the appropriate medium.

2. PURPOSE OF ELECTROPHORESIS

The purpose of Electrophoresis is the separation and identification of compounds which contain ionisable groups for example amino acids, nucleic acids, proteins, nucleotides or those which can be given weak charges by derivitisation e.g. phosphates and borates.

3. TYPES OF ELECTROPHORESIS

There are three types of electrophoresis depending on the media used.

3.1 Particle Electrophoresis

This is the migration of solid particles under the influence of electric field. The particles are observed microscopically.

3.2 Moving Boundary Electrophoresis

In this the mixture to be separated is dissolved or suspended in buffer with accurately adjusted pH.

This is then placed in a U-shaped observation cell with pure buffer layered over it (See Fig. 6.1), so that there is a boundary between pure buffer and buffer containing mixture to be separated. An electrode is then inserted into each end of the U-tube and an electric field applied.

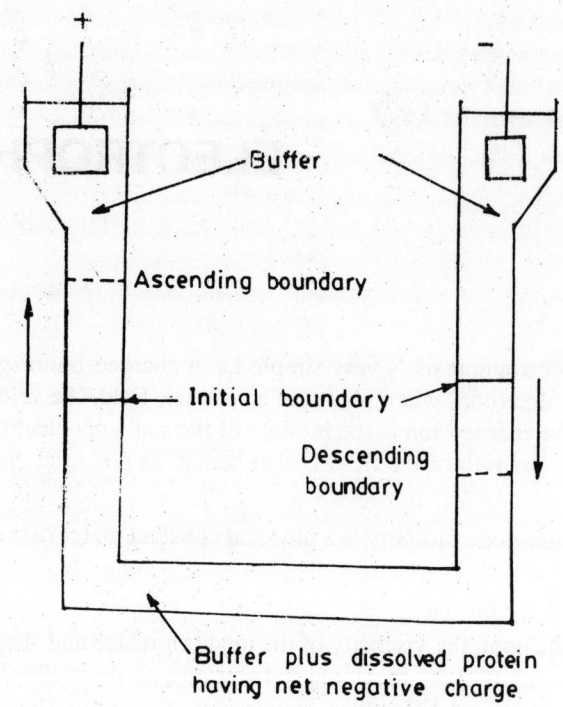

Fig. 6.1 : Moving boundary electrophoresis.

The positively charged molecules move towards cathode while the negatively charged molecules move towards the anode i.e. towards the region of the pure buffer. Consequently the refractive index at the boundary changes and this is recorded to give electrophoretic patterns called schlieren patterns that show the direction and relative rate of migration of the charged groups in the mixture.

However this form of electrophoresis suffers from a major drawback of diffusion of separated components because it is carried out in free solution.

3.3 Zone Electrophoresis

To overcome the problem of diffusion and mixing of components of the solution the solution is held in a stabilising medium such as a sheet of paper or gel. Because of the mechanical rigidity of this material, diffusion does not occur and separation is achieved in discrete zones and hence the name Zone Electrophoresis. The materials most commonly used are starch gels, paper, cellulose acetate membranes.

This has higher resolution than Moving Boundary Electrophoresis. This is because the three dimensional network of pores in such materials excludes or retards particles according to their molecular size as in Exclusion Chromatography. Hence molecules are separated on the basis of size in addition to differences in electrophoretic mobility. However, absolute electrophoretic mobility values cannot be determined because values obtained are always relative to the supporting medium.

After the run, the paper is rapidly dried in an oven. In case of a gel it is either placed in a fixative which precipitates the substances being examined with the result that the separated substances remain in their correct positions of migration or into some enzyme stain which results in the precipitation of an insoluble reaction product.

The simplest and earliest form of Zone Electrophoresis is that carried out on paper as the stabilising medium. A strip of paper is moistened with buffer, sample is applied on the paper and the paper is then sandwiched between two glass plates, (Fig. 6.2) such that each end of the paper dips into a separate beaker containing pure buffer.

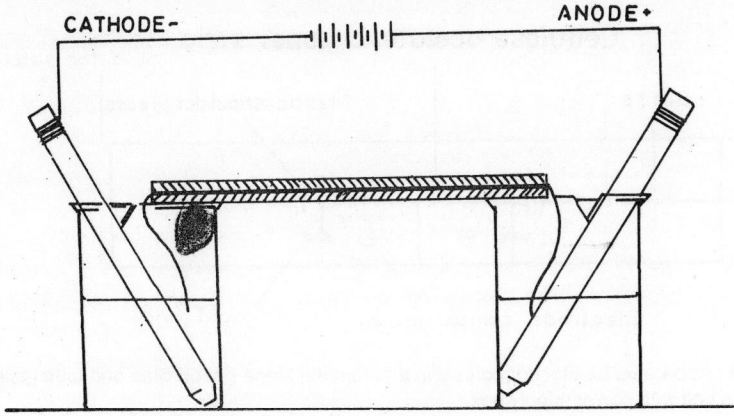

Fig. 6.2 : The simplest form of electrophoretic apparatus.

Current is then applied via a 120 volt battery and carbon electrodes dipping into each beaker. After separation, the paper is quickly dried in an oven and a locating reagent sprayed to locate the separated substances.

In the above case the buffer on the paper and beakers is the same. This is referred to as a continuous buffer system. When the beaker buffer is chemically different and has a different pH to that of the stabilising medium the system is referred to as a discontinuous buffer system. This results in faster movement and sharp resolution of zones and is now the standard procedure in starch gel electrophoresis. However the mechanism of this sharpening is not well understood. During the pasage of current electrolysis occurs at the electrodes resulting in pH changes. This is minimised by isolating the electrode in a separate compartment from that into which paper dips. These two compartments are connected by means of a paper wick, glass fiber wick or gel bridge (See Fig. 6.3).

In the case of paper electrophoresis the ends of the strip dip into the buffer and make direct connection. With CA, agar and starch gel the medium is connected by means of a further paper wick whose one end overlaps the stabilising medium by about 1cm and whose other end dips into the buffer. In all cases, the medium should be horizontal to prevent siphoning and water logging.

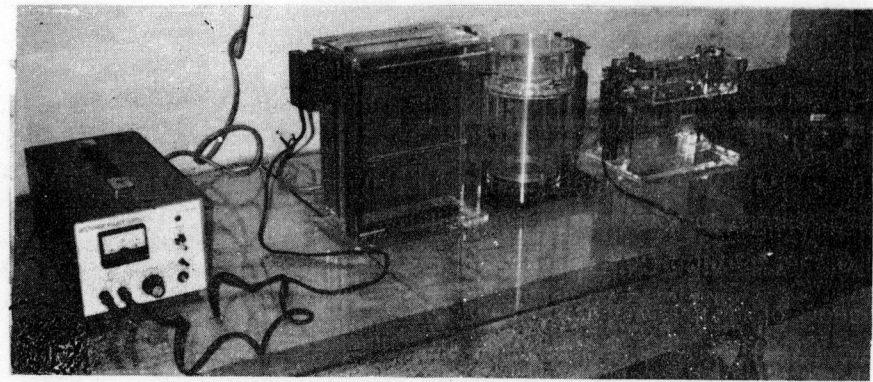

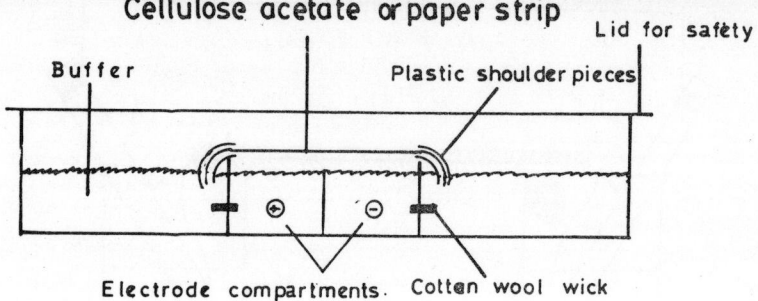

Cellulose acetate or paper strip

Fig. 6.3 : Apparatus for electrophoresis in a horizontal plane (Inset) Slab and tube gel electrophoresis unit with power supply box.

However, it has been found possible to dispense with the double buffer compartments and the paper wicks in the acrylamide gel techniques by overcoming the pH changes by using large buffer volumes or by continuously mixing and recirculating the buffer solutions.

4. FACTORS AFFECTING SPEED OF MIGRATION AND SEPARATION

4.1 Stabilising or Supporting Medium.

These are of two types:

1a. Paper, cellulose acetate, glass fibre paper, thin layer materials agar gel, single cellulose fibres. Analytical and preparative.

1b. Pevikon, starch and gypsum blocks sponge rubber. Preparative only.

2. Starch gel, acrylamide gel. Analytical and preparative

These were all originally designed for analytical purposes which require that sharp bands are formed, hence very small volumes (microlitres) are used. Subsequently it was found that the technique could be used for preparative purposes also where large volumes (in milliliters) could be separated though resolution was found to be less sharp. These are now called block techniques.

In stabilising media of group 1, separation occurs by migration in and through the liquid held stationary within the stabilising medium, on the basis of differences in charge to mass ratio of molecles as given by their electrophoretic mobilities $\mu = q / 6\pi r\eta$. Thus a large molecule with many charges may move to the same position as a small molecule with one charge. These are all relatively inert and have little effect on the compounds being separated. Paper has slight denaturing effect on proteins which results in minor tailing of the bands back towards the point of sample application. Paper is used both at high and low voltages for the separation of small molecules like amino acids for medium sized molecules like peptides and nucleotides and with low voltage only for large molecules like proteins, enzymes and nucleic acids. Thin layer materials are used for small and medium sized molecules. Gels are used exclusively for large molecules but by decreasing the pore size of the gel it can also be used for peptides and nucleotidees. Blocks are used for preparative purposes.

Due to the three dimensional network of pores formed in media of group 2, molecules are separated on the basis of differences in size due to the sieving effect of pores, as in exclusion chromatography. That is to say, ;larger molecules are progressively excluded with decreasing pore size and move faster than smaller molecules whose movement is retarded because they penetrate the gel particles. Thus molecules with similar charge to mass ratio but with different molecule size can be separated. Added to this advantage is the fact that resolution is sharper. This form of zone electrophoresis is also caled gel electrophoresis. Because of its wide applications it is worthy of deeper consideration later in the chapter.

4.2 pH

A substance can only migrate if it carries a charge, i.e. it is ionised. According to Henderson-Hasselbalch equation, the degree of ionisation of a weak acid or a weak base depends upon the pH .

$$pH = pK + \log \frac{\{unionised\}}{\{ionised\}}$$

Thus for a weak acid, for example since the rate of migration depends upon its degree of ionisation, migration will be faster at high pH values. The converse is true for weak bases. For ampholytes, migration occurs at pH values above or below the isoelectric point.

4.3 The Buffer

Buffer performs the dual functions of maintaining pH and carrying current.Current is maintained by electrolysis taking place at the electrode dipping into buffer reservoirs.

$$H_2O \xrightarrow{\text{anode}} + \tfrac{1}{2}O_2 + 2H^+ \; 2e\text{-}$$

$$2e^- + 2H_2O \xrightarrow{\text{cathode}} 2OH\text{-} + H_2 \uparrow$$

OH⁻ ions produced at the cathode cause increased dissociation of weak acid component (HA) of the buffer.

$$HA = H^+ + A^- \hspace{3cm} \dots (1)$$
$$OH^- + H^+ = H_2O \hspace{2.7cm} \dots (2)$$

The formation of H_2O in equation (2) shifts the equilibrium in equation (1) to the right. A⁻ ions migrate to the anode, combine with H⁺ ions to form HA while electrons are fed into the electric circuit. Thus most current between electrodes is conducted by the buffer and only a small component is provided by the sample ions. Therefore, the more concentrated the buffer, the slower will the other compounds move because the greater the quantity of buffer ions relative to other ions. The greater the proportion of current they carry. Also, the movement of ions surrounded by ions of opposite charge is retarded by the attraction of these ions so that a concentrated buffer further slows down migration ratio. However to compensate for this disadvantage, the zones are sharper.

Buffers are available for a whole pH range and an appropriate range can be chosen. For example proteins or other ampholytes can be separated in a pH range where they remain soluble. Thus a protein can be separated first with an alkaline buffer in which the components are all present as anions, the partially separated components can then be recovered and rerun in an acid buffer in which they exist as cations:

In addition to affecting migration rates, buffer concentrations also affect resolution of separations. In practice, invariably the buffer in the electrode compartment is more concentrated than buffer in the medium, and is often of different pH. Frequently the two buffer used are also chemically different. The net effect is to produce a voltage discontinuity at the interface of the two buffers and as this interface travels through a protein band the band becomes narrower and more compact.

Buffer ions particularly phosphates and borates bind to molecules resulting in different absolute and relative mobilities of a mixture of compounds when investigated with different buffers of the same pH and ionic strength. Phosphates are known to bind to proteins an borates to glyco-compounds. However, this is sometimes advantageous. Nutral moblecules can be separated if they can easily be converted to carry a charge. For example sugar molecules are converted to sugar borate ions by derivitisation with borate and can then be separated in borate buffers.

4.4 Voltage, Current and Heat Effects

The electrophoresis medium used as well as the buffer exert a resistance to current flow. Under a constant voltage, V in volts the resistance R ohms determines the current passed, I amperes, the consumption of W watts and the generation of heat in calories C.

$$V = I R$$

$$W = I V$$

$$C = Wt /4.18 \quad (t = seconds)$$

The rate of migration of ions increases with increase of current I. which is achieved by increasing voltage, since R for a given medium is constant.

This results in generation of heat, the resistance falls, therefore rate of migration increases. However, distillation from the warmer strip to the colder walls of the apparatus occurs, decreasing resistance. Thus it becomes imperative that either the current or voltage is stabilised with the help of a stabiliser, both will alter with time. When voltage is kept constant, current increases because resistance drops. Heating increases with continuous distillation from the strip. Tus the rate of migration increases until equilibrium. At voltages less than 100 volts (2-3 volts/cm length of the strip) and temperatures around 20°C increase in rate of migration is only slight because current increases only slightly for a 4cm wide strip. But at higher voltages, distillation is large and contains and so rate of migration varies throughout the experiment. With constant applied current, resistance and therefore, voltage falls continuously across the strip. This results in lowering of distillation keeping the rate of migration constant throughout the experiment.

When more than one strip, say two strips, are used in parellel resistance is halved and current doubled.

$$1 / R = 1/r_1 + 1/r_2$$

Since the strips are identical their resistance r and r are equal. It follows therefore,

$$1 / R = \frac{r_1 + r_2}{r_1 r_2}$$

$$\text{or } R = \frac{r_1 r_2}{r_1 + r_2}$$

$$\text{or } R = \frac{r^2}{2r}$$

$$\text{or } R = r/2$$

In general the resistance changes as $R = r/n$ and $I = nv/R$ where n is the number of strips used. To obtain the same degree and length of separation either a constant voltage must be applied or the current must be adjusted by multiplying by n.

The resistance R of the strip varies inversely with cross-sectional area of the strip or gel, a, and directly with length of strip l. That is,

$$R \, \alpha \, \frac{l}{a}$$

It follows therefore that in order to obtain reproducible results, current should be quoted as current density per centimeter width or the strip and voltage as and voltage drop per centimeter length of the strip not dipping into the buffer, as well as the temperature.

An electrophoresis unit consists of apart from the buffer compartments, support for stabilising medium, transparent insulating plates, electrodes and power supplies. For low voltage Electrophoresis (L.V.E) a maximum voltage of 300 volts while for High Voltage Electrophoresis(H.V.E.) 5000 volts can be applied.The HVE apparatus requires an additional cooling system since a great deal of heat is generated. The power supply includes constant voltage and constant amperage controls. Since both cannot operate simultaneously both a voltmeter and an ammeter covering the desired range are incorporated.

4.5 Electro-osmosis and Diffusion

Although these two factors do not directly affect the rate of migation, they adversely act upon the separation and resolution of components. When paper and water came into contact with each other, paper acquires a negative charge while water acquires a positive charge and streams towards the cathode carrying buffer and mixture components with it. In case of proteins this movement is in the opposite direction to that of migration so that they are carried back even beyond the origin and appear to have travelled in the reverse direction to that expected. Neutral molecules are also carried by the electro osmotic flow. In order to determine the true origin or the backward migratory effect these are usually also incorporated into the mixture. These include PVP, blue dextran, glucose and urea.

Diffusion causes broadening of bands, when the electric field is switched off after separation. However this problem is comparitively minor in Zone Electrophoresis and can be overlooked.

5. Types of Zone Electrophoresis

Depending on the stabilising medium used there is paper, cellulose acetate membrane and gel electrophoresis.

Paper Electrophoresis: Usually Whatman No. 1 or 3MM filter paper is used. The former is preferable although it has less wet strength than the latter. Substance separated is located by spraying locating reagents used in chromatography. Very satisfactory spots or bands are obtained. Low Voltage Paper Electrophoresis (LVPE) that is, voltages not exceeding 400 volts is used for the separation of proteins and enzymes. For the separation of smaller molecules like amino acids peptides, indoles, phenols, purines pyrimidines. High voltage paper electrophoresis (HVPE) is used. It has the additional advantages of high speed and better resolution. Adsorption of molecules resulting in tailing of samples occurs in paper electrophoresis but this can be reduced by using buffers more alkaline than isoelectric point of sample. A small amount of denaturation also occurs so that a pure white background is rarely obtained.

Cellulose Acetate Membrane (CAM) Electrophoresis: CAM has a continuous microporous structure and so has certain advantages over paper electrophoresis. There is very little adsoption resulting in sharp separations of well defined bands, greatly improving the accuracy of quantitative determinations. CAM can be rendered translucent by treatment with whitemor oil -120 facilitating quantification. CAM can be cut into sections and dissolved in solvents making spectrophotometric estimations possible. Since it has a low background count it is good for separations of radio labelled substances and so radiological detection of separated compounds is less hindered.

6. GEL ELECTROPHORESIS

Electrophoretic separations on paper, cellulose acetate and agar are based on a simple electrophoretic effect namely the migration of ions under the influence of an electric current. In general the medium acts as an inert support for buffer in which the separation occurs but if the medium doesexert any effect it is often adverse eg, the slight denaturing of proteins by paper causing tailing. With the advent of starch gel electrophoresis the converse was the case.

Not only did the gel affect finer separations; but the components of the mixture migrated through the pore structure of the gel which acted as a molecular sieve so that molecules of the same charge to mass ratio would separate if their molecular sizes were sufficiently different. The extreme example is of the single α_2 globulin band from paper electrophoresis which was resolved into about 10 sub-bands after Gel Electrophoresis.

Subsequent to the use of starch gels, synthetic gels began to be produced from organic monomers which were co-polymerised with another monomer in the presence of a catalyst. Use of these in gel electrophoresis showed a number of advantages over starch gel. Among these are, ease of preparation of the gel, relative inertness of the gel components and quicker running time. However, the greatest advantage of the technique is that the gel can be tailored so that the pore size can be varied in a known manner. Increase in gel concentration produces a decrease in pore size so that molecules of decreasing molecular size are excluded (as in Exclusion Chromatography). This way larger but less interesting molecules are screened out.

Such synthetic gels include dextran, agarose and polyacrylamide gels.

6.1 Dextran gels

These are obtained by cross-linking the polysacharide dextran with epichlorohydrin and are sold under the trade name Sephadex. These can separate molecules with molecular weights between 200,000 - 800,000 Daltons.

6.2 Agarose gels

Sold under the trade name sepharose, they contain alternating residues of D-ga;lactose and 3,6-anhydro-L-galactose. It is a natural linear polysaccharide derived from the agar of *Gelidium amansii*. Gels are prepared by dissolving the dry polymer in boiling water and cooling the mixture to room temperature. Gelation occurs at 45°C or lower. The highly porous yet rigid gel that forms at concentrations as low as 0.2% has been attributed to an uncrosslinked network of double strands of polymer rich in hydrogen bonding. The gel forms a porous network with pores large enough to allow even the largest molecules to pass unimpeded. Thus the sieving property of the gel is not used at all. It merely acts as a stabilising medium while particles are separated according to charge to mass ratio. Agarose extends the useful range of electrophoresis to include the largest molecules, and supramolecular complexes. e.g. many viruses, enzyme complexes, lipoprpteins and nucleic acids all of which are beyond the largest usable pore size with polyacrylamide gel electrophoresis, approximately 500 A in a 2.6% gel. In general a 0.5% agarose gel may be substituted for cellulose acetate or paper strips for better separations of small as well as large molecules.

6.3 Polyacrylamide Gel Electrophoresis (PAGE)

PAGE is similar to Agarose Gel Electrophoresis except that the gel pores are small enough to slow down the large proteins so that strict separation by charge to mass ratio is modified by a sieving effect. Polyacrylamide gels are generated by free radical polymerisation of acrylamide monomer, $CH_2 = CH-CO-NH_2$, and the cross-linking co-monomer N, N, N - methylene - bis-acrylamide, $CH_2 = CH — CO — NH — CH2 NH — CO — CH = CH_2$.

The polymerisation reaction is initiated by a catalyst redox system which furnishes free radicals. The most commonly used catalyst - initiator system utilises the tertiary amine TEMED. N, N, N' - tetramethylethylene diamine as catalyst and ammonium persulfate as initiator which generates oxygen free radicals. The pore size can be varied by varying the percentage of acrylamide as given in Table 6.1.

7. Gradient Electrophoresis, SDS Electrophoresis

Gradient electrophoresis : A pore gradient gel - one in which an increasing concentration of polyacrylamide decreases the size of pores in the direction of electrophoretic mobility. This can be used to separate native proteins by size rather than charge. When an electric field is applied to a pore gradient gel molecules begin moving at a speed determined by charge. But as the pore size decreases, the larger molecules begin to slow down and are finally immobilised at the point where the pores are so small that the molecules can no longer squeeze through. Since the leading edge of a particular band of

Table 6.1: Correlation between acrylamide concentration and pore size.

Acrylamide (%)	Radius of pore size (Å)	Molecular Weight
2.5	25	-
3.75	-	10^6
5	18	-
7.5	15	3×10^5
10.0	13	-
20.0	10	-
15-30	-	10^4
30-35	5	-

molecules stops before the tailing edge, the tailing edge has a chance to catch up and a narrow band is formed. Smaller molecules even if they are weakly charged and move slowly, have a chance to migrate past the larger ones, until they too reach a they are immobilised . Because of its sharply stacked bands, gradient electrophoresis is one of the highest resolution methods.

SDS Electrophoresis : Proteins can also be separated on the basis of size alone if they sodium dodecyl sulphate (SDS) which binds to molecules converting them to rod like molecules masking their native charge with its own negative charge. When subjected to PAGE the proteins which are now equal in charge density are separated purely according to size by molecular sieving effect of the gel.

In SDS PAGE migration rate correlates quite accurately with molecular weight, and the method is used frequently for molecular weight determination. Treatment of proteins with SDS and a reducing agent changes their compact three dimensional shape into rod like structures. Since the SDS molecules bind to polypeptides with a constant weight ratio the charge per unit weight is constant and electrophoretic mobility becomes a function of molecular weight. The technique of SDS PAGE has been widely used for the determination of molecular weights of unknown proteins by comparing their relative electrophoretic mobility to standard proteins of known molecular weights see Table 6.2.

8. TWO DIMENSIONAL ELECTROPHORESIS

This technique involves a combination of two different electrophoretic separations in single dimension: The first dimensional separation is usually carried out in cylindrical gels. This gel is then placed on top of a slab and serves as the sample for the second dimensional separation. Ideally, each dimension should fractionate the protein mixture according to their different physical and chemical properties.

9. NUCLEIC ACID ELECTROPHORESIS

Nucleic acids which are invariable in charge to mass ratio, are propelled with equal velocity in an electric field, but can be separated according to size by selecting a gel which will sieve the molecules. Agarose gels are used to sieve very large molecules such

Table 6.2 Composition of SDS-PAGE Standards.

Product Description	Protein	Molecular Weight
SDS-PAGE standards	Lysozyme	14,400
Low Molecular weight	Soybean trypsin inhibitor	21,500
	Carbonic anhydrase	31,000
	Ovalbumin	45,000
	Bovine serum albumin	66,200
	Phosphorylase B	92,500
SDS PAGE Standards	Ovalbumin	45,000
High Molecular Weight	Bovine serum albumin	66,200
	Phosphorylase	B92,500
	- galactosidase	1,16,250
	Myosin	2,00,000

as intact pieces of DNA or RNA, while polyacrylamide gels can be used for separation of smaller RNA or DNA fragments. Techniques of agarose and polyacrylamide gel electrophoresis are used extensively in the analysis of the size structure and function of DNA and RNA molecules. In particular recent developments in recombinant DNA techniques, restriction fragment mapping and nucleic acid sequencing have utilised gel electrophoresis as a sensitive analytical tool. Restriction enzymes which cut DNA molecules at specific sequences, are used to generate defined fragments of DNA whose size is determined by gel electrophoresis. The technique is very sensitive allowing the detection of les than 10 nanograms of material per band upon staining with 1 μg/ml ethidium bromide. Choice of the proper gel medium is determined by the molecular weight range of the molecules to be separated. Nucleic acids have well defined molecular weights which vary from 350 daltons for a single base to over 33×10 daltons, the size of the phage lambda genome. Agarose gels have proven to be an ideal medium for the separation of large restriction fragments, while polyacrylamide and agarose acrylamides gels are used widely for the separation of smaller restriction fragments and RNA molecules.

Several new methods of rapidly sequencing nucleic acids have been introduced which allow the nucleotide sequence of DNA and RNA fragments to be read directly from the gel. These methods involve the use of high percentage polyacrylamide gels capable of resolving fragments which vary length by only one nucleotide. In gels prepared for sequencing and molecular weight determinations it is necessary to keep the molecules in a fully denatured form, since variations in secondary structures lead to variations in electrophoretic mobility. The commonly used denaturing gels contain either 6-8 M urea or 99% formamide. Under these conditions the electrophoretic mobility is independent of base composition and secondary structures; all single stranded molecules of the same length migrate identically. Due to ionic impurities in urea and formamide which lead to high conductivity, it is necessary to deionize them before gel preparation.

Thus we find and further see that gel electrophoresis is an extraordinarily flexible method for separation and analysis of proteins nucleic acids and other charged molecules, which are propelled through a porous gel and are separated by their different electrophoretic mobilities. Variations in the gel and buffer make it possible to separate molecules not only according to charge but also according to molecular weight isoelectric point (Isoelectric focussing) and biospecific affinity (Immunoelectrophoresis).

10. ISOELECTRIC FOCUSSING

Isoelectric focussing takes advantage of the fact that each amphoteric molecule or zwitterion has a different pH at which it is electrically neutral its isoelectric point , pI. These amphoteric molecules are focussed at thier isoionic points under voltage and pH gradients generated within the gel with a low pH at the anode to a highl pH at the cathode (See Fig. 6.4). Voltage gradient causes differential migration of charged species while pH gradients influence the type of charge on the zwittrion. A zwitterion is a dipolar ion which at its isoelectric point, pI has no net charge. When an electric field is applied the positively charged molecules move towards the cathode while the negatively charged molecules move towards the anode. When each molecule reaches neutrality at its pI, the

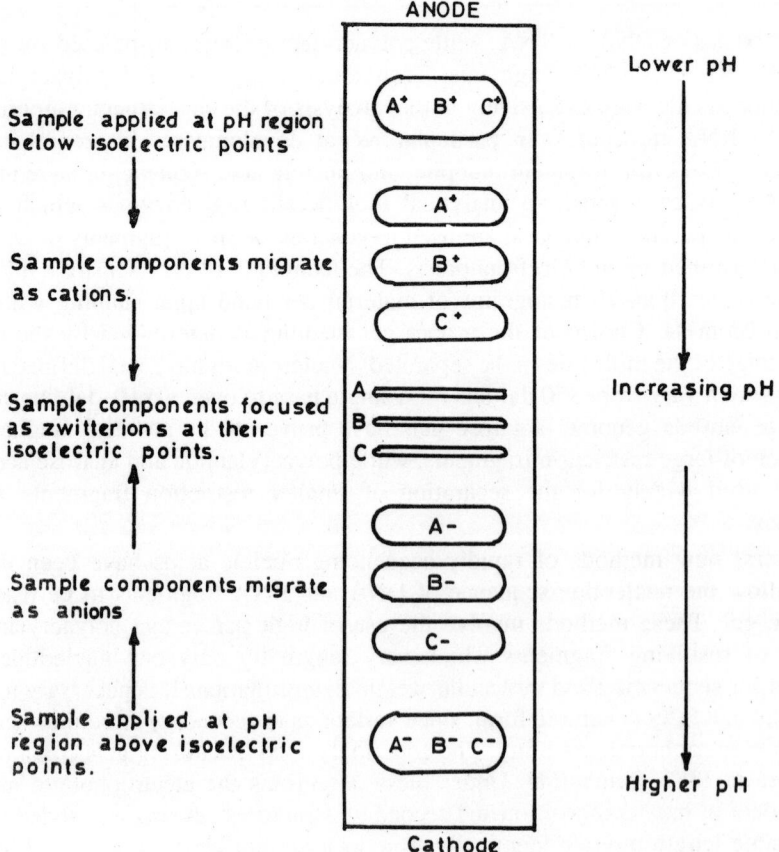

Fig. 6.4 : The Principle of isoelectric focussing.

pH at which there is no net charge on the molecule, it loses its electrophoretic mobility and becomes focussed in a narrow zone. Diffusion is offset by the electric field and so the bands do not broaden.

The pH gradient itself is generated by a mixture of carrier ampholytes that come to rest in order of its pI when subjected to an electric field, and each of which maintains a local pH corresponding to its pI by virtue of its strong buffering capacity. Isoelectric focussing can be used analytically to determine isoelectric points, to assay the purity of a sample or to test its composition. It can also be used preparatively to obtain a highly purified fraction.

11. IMMUNOELECTROPHORESIS

The separating power of a gel can be greatly enhanced by combining it with techniques based on the ability of a ligand such as an antibody, to precipitate a complex molecule from a complex mixture. Immunoelectrophoresis is based on electrophoresis of antigenic proteins into an antibody containing gel which results in the precipitation of antigen - antibody complexes.

12. ISOTACHOPHORESIS

In conventional electrophoresis the electrophoretic system consists of two electrodes which are connected by a conducting medium called electrolyte. The electrolyte is often the negatively charged glycinate ion buffered to pH 8.6 with Tris. Since there is one continuous conducting medium between anode and cathode, the field strength E, through the system is constant. Since $v = \mu E$, the velocity of an ion placed in this system will be proportional to its net mobility ($v \alpha \mu$). As a result, an ion with a high net mobility can be separated from an ion with a low net mobility. The separation thus results from ions moving at different velocities in a continuous electrolyte system.

In a discontinuous electrolyte system, two different electrolytes are used. One electrolyte contains a high net mobility ion and the other contains a low net mobility ion. The two electrolytes are called the "leading electrolyte" and the "terminating electrolyte " respectively. For example, if the leading electrolyte is Tris/Cl and the terminating electrolyte is Tris/Glycinate, the negatively charged chloride ion has greater net mobility than the glycinate ion. Tris is the counter ion which gives the highest possible bufferring capacity in the working pH range. The leading electrolyte is in contact with the anode (Fig. 6.5) and the terminating electrolyte is in contact with the cathode.

The leading and terminating electrolytes can also be positively charged ions in which case the leading electrolyte is in contact with the cathode.

Let us call the ion in the leading electrolyte L⁻, and the ion in the terminating electrolyte T. Suppose that we have two sample ions A⁻ and B⁻, which we put at the boundary between the two electrolytes. The net mobility of A⁻ is higher than that of B, and the net mobilities of A and B are betwen those of L⁻ and T⁻ that is,

$$\mu_L \text{-} > \mu_A \text{-} > \mu_B \text{--} > \mu_T \text{-}$$

When an electric field is applied, the negatively charged ions begin to move towards the anode. As they do so, they arrange themselves in order of net mobility. Since there is initially a uniform field strength over the zone containing both A and B ions, the ions start to separate within that zone according to the equation $v = \mu E$. After a time, we have

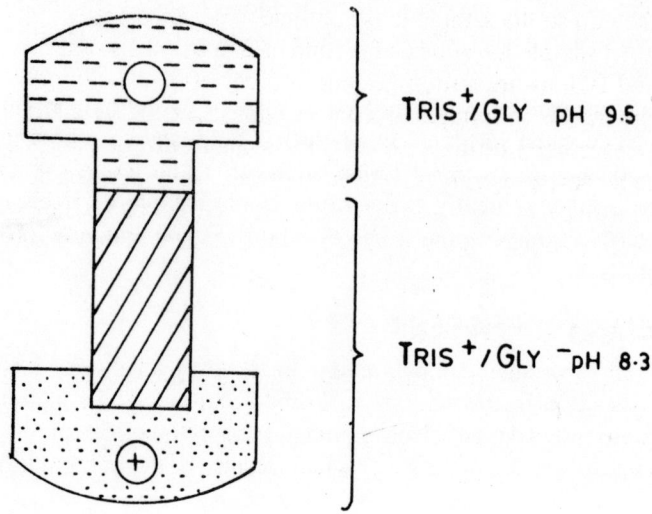

Fig. 6.5 : Discontinous electrolyte system.

one zone containing only A ions and the counter ion, one zone containing only B ions and the counter ion, and in between them a mixed zone which contains both A and B ions (Fig. 6.6a).

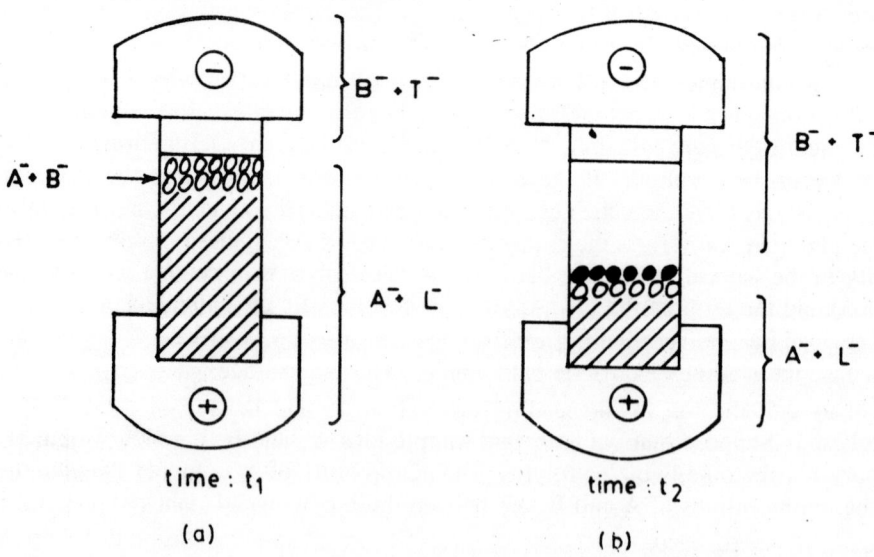

Note :- The sample components are conducting the current

No background electrolyte

Fig. 6.6 : Isotachophoresis

The leading electrolyte, sample ions and terminating electrolyte all travel towards the anode. As they do so the sample ions continue to separate until, at equilibrium there are just two distinct sample ion zones, of A⁻ and of B ions. At equilibrium, the two zones containing A⁻ and B⁻ ions are still migrating in order of their net mobilities. In the ion "train" each zone travels in immediate contact with its neighbours and therefore at the same velocity; the velocity of these zones is the same as that of the leading electrolyte. This is why, the technique is called isotachophoresis. Iso = same tacho = velocity. It is important to point out that the sample components are conducting the current. Unlike conventional electrophoresis, there is no background electrolyte, which means that in each zone we find only the sample component and the counter ion.

13. STAINING AND FIXATION.

The separated components are localised by staining with specific dyes. Quantitative measurements can be made by cutting out the portion of gel containing the separated fraction, dissolving the gel in a suitable solvent and quantifying it by spectrophotometric measurement since the dye - macromolecule complex has a λ_{max}. See Table 6.3.

Table 6.3

Stain	max	Use
Amido black 10B Buffalo Black, Naphthalene Black 10B	620	General protein stain
Coomassie Brilliant Blue R-250	590	General protein stain more sensitive than Amido black
Coomassie Brilliant Blue G-250	595	General protein stain
Acacian Blue	630	Glycoprotein
Methylene Blue	665	RNA, RNase
Methylene Green	635	Native DNA acidic or neutral tracking dye
Fast Green FCF	610	Protein stain
Basic Fuchsin	550	Glycoprotein Nucleic acid Sialic acid rich glycoproteins
Pyronin Y	510	RNA, acidic tracking dye
Bromophenol blue	595	Neutral and alkaline tracking dye
Crocein scarlet	505	Immunoelectrophoresis
Ethidium bromide		Fluorimetric detection of DNA

Alternatively, the method of "Blotting " capillary and electrophoretic transfer to derivatized cellulose paper is used for detection and analysis of electrophoretically resolved molecules. Transferred nucleic acid fragments are easily detected by hybridisation using labelled DNA or RNA probes. Transferred antigens, antibodies, hormones receptors and glycoproteins can also be detected with the appropriate probes followed by fluorescent, enzyme substrate or autoradiographic assay.

After staining, gels are fixed in one of the two fixatives listed below. Following fixation permanent records of gels are kept on 35 mm photographic films. Stains involving a fluorescent reaction cannot be fixed and must be photographed through a yellow filter. The "alcohol gel wash" fixative not only fixes the stain but also toughens the gel and helps bleach out some of the background. In some cases it also dissolves the stained precipitate and so glycerine and water fixative is used.

A : Alcohol gel wash

Ethanol	.....	1000 ml
Acetic acid	.....	400 ml
Glycerine	.....	200 ml
Water	.....	800 ml

B : Glycerine and water

Glycerine	.....	500 ml
Water	.....	500 ml

14. APPLICATIONS

With the advancement towards molecular biology, electrophoresis and particularly gel electrophoresis is very widely used for separation and identification of macromolecules e.g. nucleic acids, amino acids, enzymes and proteins. Gradient gel electrophoresis provides the advantage of improved resoltuion and zone sharpening. These properties of the technique have been put to use for the detection of certain physiological disorders which are manifested as production of a different kind of enzyme or protein as compared to normal e.g. the differences in the proteins present in the sputum of normal and asthmatic individuals or differences in haptoglobins in Alzheimer's disease.

In addition to helping in diagnosis of clinical disorders, Gel electrophoresis can be used to identify mutants of microorganisms. A "mutant" is an individual with a different genetif make-up as compared to the "wild type". Due to the small size of DNA of microorganisms it is possible to break it up using "restriction enzymes". These enzymes cleave DNA at very specific points giving rise to polynucleotides of specific chain length. This is then run on a gel so that bands of different polynucleotide lengths are obtained. All cells of wild type will have their DNA broken up into similar number of polynucleotides having similar chain length. The mutant DNA will show a different number of polynucleotides. This difference is observed by hybridisation with "Probe" which is radiolabelled DNA broken up by the same restriction enzymes. The technique is called "restriction analysis" and is a fool proof technique to search out a mutant organism.

7

X-RAY MICROANALYSIS

X-ray microanalysis makes it possible for chemical analysis to be performed on biological tissue within very small and well-defined regions of the specimen. All elements from Na to U can be detected while observing the specimen in the electron microscope. As little as 10^{-17} to 10^{-18} g of an element can be detected. It is used in such diverse scientific areas as metallurgy, physics, electronics, minerology, environmental pollution, geology and lately in pathology, zoology, biochemistry and other biological fields.

1. PRINCIPLE

Atoms when struck by electrons from an external source, yield X-rays which are characteristic of those atoms and are used to identify and quantify the elements present. The method combines electron microscopy and X-ray spectroscopy. During electron microscopical observation of a specimen, the sample is bombarded with high energy electrons which generate characteristic and continuous background X-rays in the irradiated area of the sample. If the exciting electron beam is focussed to a diameter of 100 nm on an ultrathin section of same thickness, a slightly conical electron probe of this size is formed within the specimen and X-ray emission is restricted to this probed area. Thus we can observe the specimen in the electron microscope, select the feature of interest, focus the electron beam onto this and record the generated X-ray spectrum.

X-ray Production : In Fig. 7.1, the nucleus comprising neutrons and protons is surrounded by orbital electrons distributed in different energy levels K, L, M etc. X-ray microanalysis is based upon the excitation of these electrons to produce an emitted X-ray spectrum which is characteristic of the element concerned. If one of the orbital electrons is removed from its energy level by an incident electron then the atom is said to be in an excited state. When this occurs, an electron from a higher energy state will fall down into the gap to stabilise the atom. Because of the difference in potential energy levels the excess energy is emitted during this electron transition as an X-ray photon. Thus if an electron in the K-shell is removed, a second electron from the L-shell may instantaneously replace it, thus giving off its excess energy as a photon of energy $E_L - E_K$ generally called E_α radiation. Now the filling of the vacancy in the K shell by an electron from the L-shell will also produce a vacancy in the L shell which in turn may be filled with one from the M shell and so on each with the production of X-ray photons of energies determined by the orbital energies. Thus a single ionisation can give rise to a whole spectrum of characteristic X-rays and this energy spectrum identifies the atom.

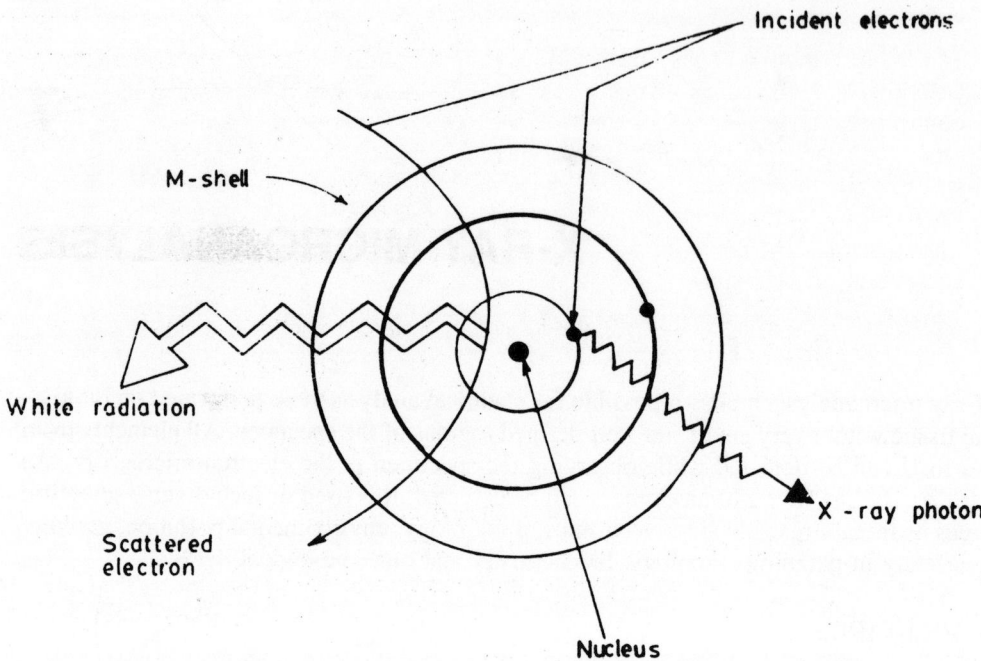

Fig. 7.1 : Simple schematic representation of an atom showing x-ray production.

If a primary electron beam, instead of interfering with the orbital electrons to produce characteristic X-rays, may interact with the nucleus. As the incoming electron beam is decelerated by the field of nuclear charge it radiates energy which can be anything from the maximum originally carried by the electrons to a small fraction of it. Fig. 7.2 shows the energy spectrum produced by this effect with the maximum energy

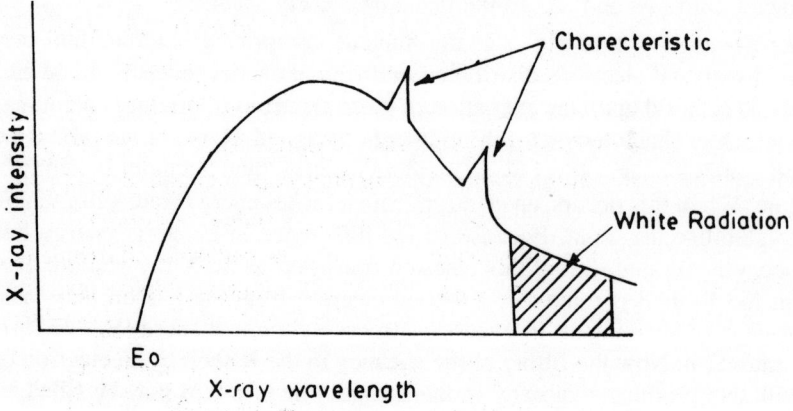

Fig. 7.2 : X-ray-continuum.

being that of the primary electron beam E. This general spectrum is called "X-ray continuum" or "continuous radiation" or "white radiation" or "Bremsstrahlung". It forms the background upon which the characteristic X-ray lines are superimposed at specific wavelengths or energies.

White radiation forms a basic limitation to the ability to detect a characteristic "line" and it is considered as X-ray noise. It is however useful in calculating elemental concentrations.

2. Instrumentation

For viewing biological material, there are two methods. Thin specimens are viewed in transmission and bulk specimens are viewed by reflection. Instrumental arrangements are acordingly of two types.

   (a) Scanning electron microscope + X-ray detection system.

   (b) Transmission electron microscope + X-ray detection system.

X-ray detection systems used generally are also of two types viz. wavelength dispersive crystal spectrometers and energy dispersive solid state detectors. Wavelength dispersive crystal spectrometers work on the principle that of the X-rays leaving the specimen, a narrow cone falls on a curved crystal and a fraction of this signal is reflected into a detector which is usually a gas flow, or sealed, proportional counter. In the detector the X-rays are converted to electrical signals, amplified and transferred to a multichannel analyser. The individual channels are calibrated by energy and the channel number or energy position gives qualitative analytical information. The fraction of signal which is reflected depends upon the the crystal's ability to "diffract" a particular wavelength maximally and is governed by Bragg's law which states that for crystals

$$2d \, \sin\theta \ = n\lambda$$

where n is an integer, λ is the X-ray wavelength maximally diffracted d is the lattice spacing of the crystal and θ is the angle of incidence (and of reflection) of the X-ray beam at the crystal. Every element in the periodic table has X-ray lines corresponding to characteristic wavelength (λ) values. A crystal having value (wavelength maximally diffracted) same as λ value of X-rays emitted by element, the crystal not only detects this element but also quantifies it. In order to extend the range of elements detected, a number of crystals are incorporated in the instrument. All the crystals have different "d" values or lattice spacings, so that for the same θ range the wavelength (λ) range is enlarged thereby covering a number of elements.

The energy dispersive solid state detector can detect all X-ray energies leaving the specimen at once unlike the crystal spectrometer which can detect only one at a time. The solid state detector provides an energy spectrum of all elements analysed simultaneously. Here, the incoming X-rays are sorted and analysed by their energies and consists of a liquid nitrogen cooled Si/Li semiconductor.

Fig. 7.3 illustrates the incorporation of crystal detectors or solid state detectors or both at appropriate positions with respect to the electron microscope either in the scanning mode or transmission mode. In scanning electron microscope the detectors can be easily brought close to the specimen for greater sensitivity.

Both one dimensional and two dimensional analysis can be performed with scanning electron microscope. For two dimensional analysis, the detector is set so as to collect X-

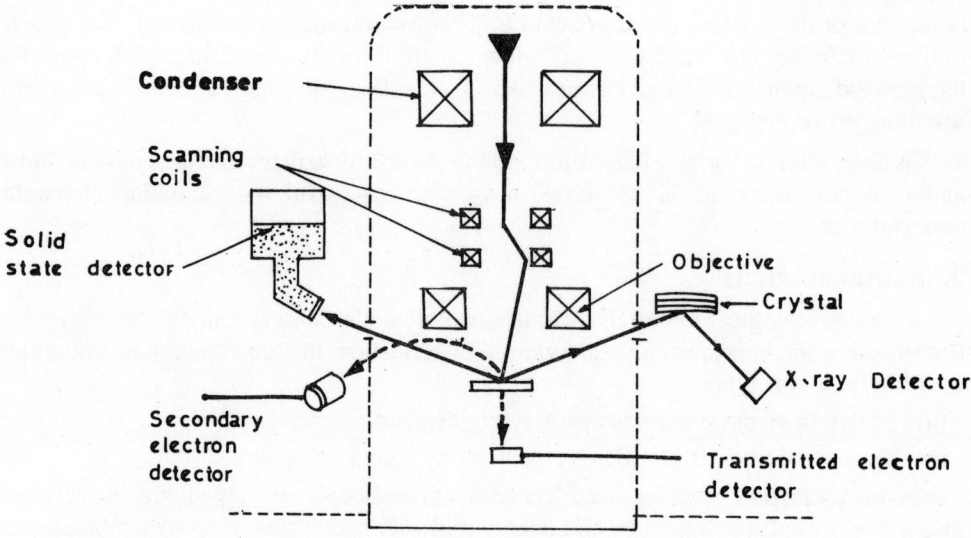

Fig. 7.3 : Schematic representation of a scanning electron microscope incorporating X-ray microanalysis.

rays from only a particular element of interest and then the focussed electron beam is made to scan the specimen. The X-ray signal from the detector is displayed on a cathode ray oscilloscope by synchronising with the electron beam raster. For one dimensional analysis i.e. a line trace, the output is fed in to a chart recorder so that changes in elemental content can be monitored across that line in the specimen. To analyse a particular area of interest a static probe is directed over that area and X-ray emission analysed over a period of time (Fig. 7.4).

Almost any electron microscope can thus be converted to an X-ray analyser by attacking a suitable detector to the specimen region. This idea was first given by Castaign in 1949 and in 1968, the first electron microscope with X-ray analyser was constructed.

3. APPLICATIONS

Several problems can be tackled using this technique.

(i) Natural elemental composition of tissues can be demonstrated by analysis of normal physiological levels after appropriately preparing the specimen for analysis.

(ii) Accidentally introduced foreign material e.g. toxic chemicals can be located and identified within the tissue.

(iii) Deliberately introduced elements eg. by administration of drugs can be traced throughout the tissue and related to morphological changes which follow due to this.

(iv) Histochemistry and immunochemistry of living systems can be studied *in situ* by analysis of biochemical events.

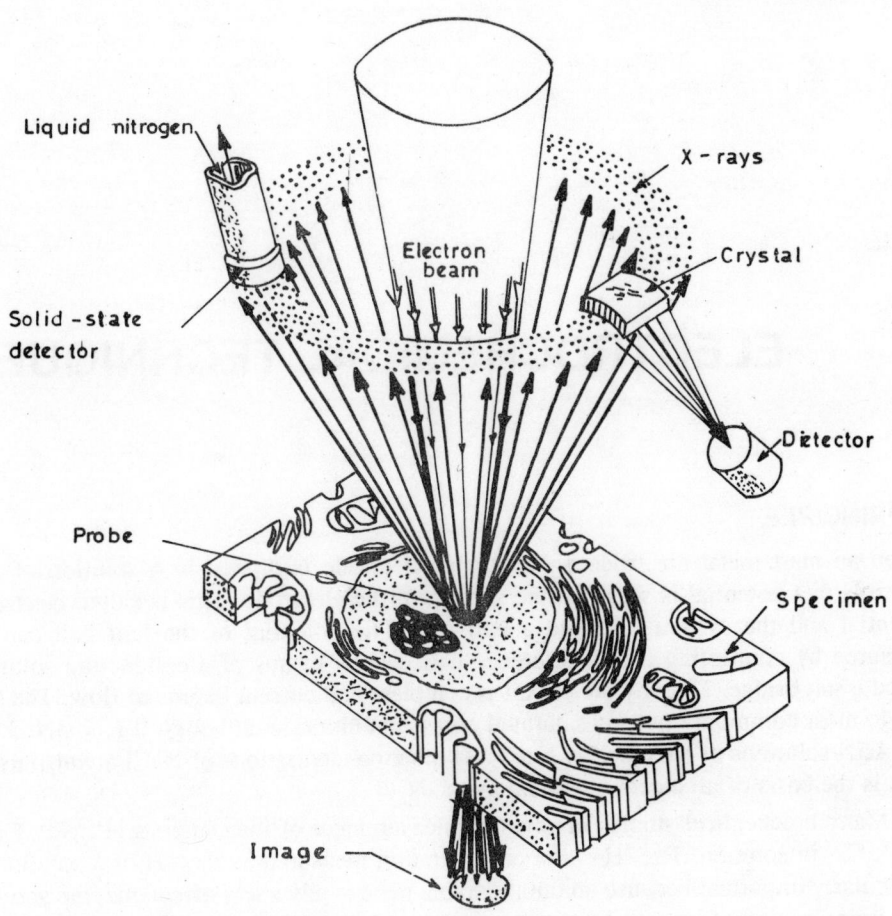

Fig. 7.4 : Schematic representation of x-ray microanalysis of thin spections with transmission electron microscopy.

8

ELECTROCHEMICAL TECHNIQUES

1. PRINCIPLE

When an inert metal electrode eg. platinum electrode is dipped in a solution of an electrolyte, a potential is set up at the surface of the electrode. This is called electrode potential and the system is called a half cell. The potential of the half cell can be measured by connecting it to a reference half cell by means of a conducting solution called a salt bridge. Thereby the circuit is complete and current begins to flow. The salt bridge most commonly used is saturated potassium chloride, although 0.1 N, 3N, 3.5N and 4.5N solutions of KCl, 0.15N NaCl and other concentrations of NaCl are also used. This is the basis of all electrochemical methods.

Many biochemical studies involve the measurement of ions such as H^+, Na^+, Ca^{2+}, NH_4^+, Cl^- in solution. The H^+ ion concentration measured as the pH of a solution is particularly important because an unfavourable pH can adversely affect enzyme activity of a living system. Denatured enzymes result in a complete breakdown of metabolism thereby making such studies impossible. pH is measured using glass electrodes but rough estimates can also be made using pH sensitive dyes which change colour at specific pH. Electrodes measuring the concentration of other ions are called ion selective electrodes in general.

Many biological processes e.g. respiration and photosynthesis convert one form of energy into another as per the requirement of the cell. For example, respiration converts chemical energy into a more readily utilisable form while photosynthesis converts solar energy into chemical energy so that it can be trapped inside the cell. These processes involve electron carriers which bring about oxidation - reduction reactions within the cell. The ease with which a compound can accept or donate an electron is expressed by its oxidation - reduction (redox) potential. i.e. the potential arising from two ions of the same element in different states of oxidation eg. Fe^{2+}/Fe^{3+} (in contrast to one between element and its ion - electrode potential). The redox potential can be most accurately measured elctrochemically using a platinum electrode, although rough estimates can be made using redox dyes.

Just as H^+ ion concentration within the cell is of great importance, dissolved oxygen concentration changes within the cell are very valuable for biochemical studies since oxygen utilisation or evolution is fundamental to many biological processes. Oxygen electrodes which measure dissolved oxygen as current flowing between a platinum and a silver-silver chloride electrode immersed in a saturated KCl solution which has been equilibrated with dissolved oxygen in an unknown solution by diffusion across a semi-permeable membrane. The current results from oxygen uptake of electrons at the platinum electrode's surface after the electrode is polarised using a direct current voltage.

2. THE pH METER

pH is defined as $-\log_{10} [H^+]$. A pH measurement is an indirect measurement of the hydrogen ion activity. The hydrogen ion activity coefficient approaches unity in very dilute solutions. Therefore, this activity measurement can be a workable approximation for concentration. A pH value of 0-7 represents acidic range and from 7-14 alkaline range.

A pH meter consists of two electrodes - an indicator electrode sensitive to hydrogen ion concentration and a reference electrode whose potential remains constant. When these two electrodes are dipped in the test solution, the potential of the electrode chain that develops is measured with a galvanometer calibrated for a pH scale. The whole unit is called a pH meter.

Reference electrode: This is usually a saturated calomel electrode (Fig. 8.1). It consists of a saturated solution of KCl in contact with a paste of mercurous chloride (calomel Hg Cl) and mercury. This reference half cell can be written as :

$$Hg \qquad Hg_2 \quad Cl_2 \quad saturated \qquad test\ solution$$
$$KCl$$

The double lines indicate the presence of a salt bridge. The chloride ions become saturated with mercury at the surface of the mercury. Under these conditions the electrode produces a constant reference potential to which the indicator electrode potential is compared. For proper operation it is best to keep the electrode tip immersed in the electrolyte. The bridge salt solution should be the same as the electrode's electrolyte. The calomel electrode is separated from the KCl salt bridge by a porous ceramic plug which reduces back diffusion and contamination.

An alternative to the calomel electrode is the silver - silver chloride electrode. It consists of a silver wire on which silver chloride is deposited. This is then dipped in a chloride solution e.g. KCl

$$Ag \qquad AgCl \quad KCl \qquad test\ solution$$

Historically, the most important reference electrode is the standard hydrogen electrode. It consists of an inert metal electrode e.g. platinum immersed in a solution of fixed concentration of HCl and in which pure hydrogen gas is bubbled at one atmosphere pressure establishing the <u>following</u> equilibrium

$$1/2 \qquad H_2 \qquad\qquad H^+ + e^-$$

The platinum electrode is covered by aS surface catalyst such as platinum black or palladium black, which reduces the energy barier, increases the equilibrium pressure of hydrogen and makes the electrode reversible in response to hydrogen ion. However, this electrode is highly inconvenient to use because the hydrogen gas has to be generated at a constant pressure and must be oxygen free and the platinum black is also readily contaminated. In practice, therefore oxidation reduction potentials are expressed relative

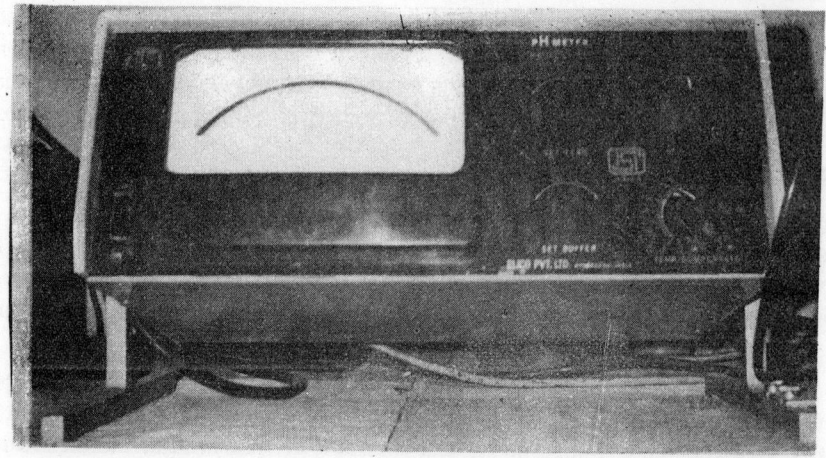

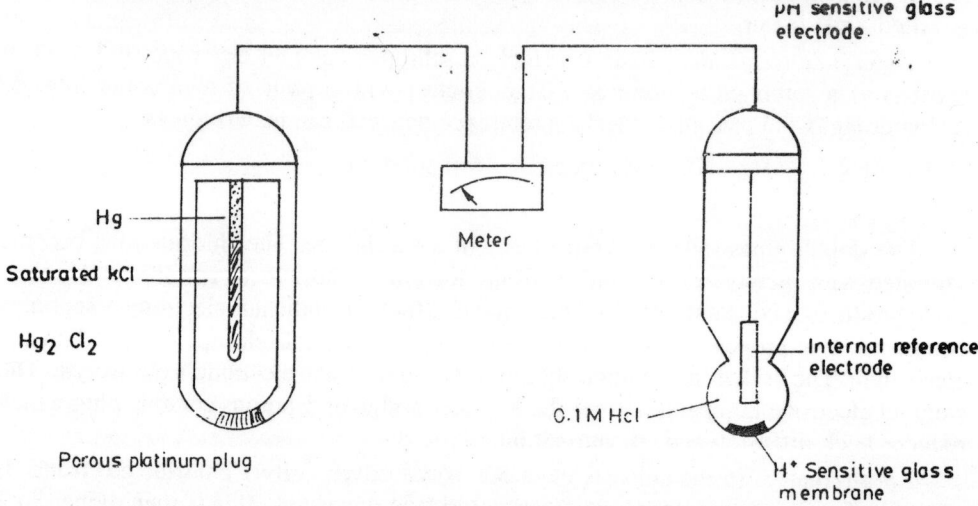

Fig. 8.1 : Schematic pH system (inset) A pH Meter.

to the standard hydrogen electrode whose potential is arbitrarily assigned as 0.0000V, other reference electrodes generally calomel electrodes are used.

Indicator electrode: Glass electrode is the most commonly used indicator electrode (Fig. 8.1). It consists of an internal electrode of the silver-silver chloride type immersed in 0.1M HCl inside a glass bulb. The glass bulb is made of thin glass membrane (0.03 - 0.1 mm thickness). The glass is of special type which develops a potential difference when ionic solutions of different pH are present on its two sides. Thus or its one side is the test solution while on the other is 0.1M HCl of known pH. Glass consists of a silicate network amongst which are metal ions coordinated to oxygen atoms and the metal ions exchange with H^+ of the external test solution. Ion exchange occurs on the hydrated layer formed on the glass surface which is of 50-100 Å thickness. When the H^+ ion concentration changes in the external solution, the accompanying change in potential n the outisde surface of the bulb is transmitted to the inside surface which in turn is transmitted to the internal silver-silver chloride electrode. This however measures only hydrogen ion activity and not hydrogen ion concentration. The glass electrode acts like a battery whose voltage depends on the H^+ ion activity of the solution in which it is immersed. The size of the potential (E) due to H^+ ions is given by the equation:

$$E = 2.303 \ \frac{RT}{F} \ \log \frac{[H^+]i}{[H^+]o}$$

where [H]i and [H]o is the molar concentrations of H ions inside and outside the glass electrode. In practice, [H]i is fixed and is generally equal to 10since the electrode contains 0.1M HCl. Since pH = -log [H], it follows that the potential developed is directly proportional to the pH of the solution outside the electrode.

Glass electrodes are particularly useful since there is no interference from components of the solution. The mineral composition of glass is critical. The general formula of all types of glass electrodes includes 72%, SiO, 6% Cao$_2$. 21% Na$_2$ O, 1% Al$_2$O$_3$ produces a good pH sensitive glass membrane with little metal response. The concentration of oxides of sodium and aluminium are varied to make different types of electrodes which include the pH type, the cation type and the sodium type.

The two electrodes namely the reference and indicator electrodes are connected to a galvanometer calibrated for a pH scale which measures the change in potential between them.

3. THE OXYGEN ELECTRODE

There are several types of oxygen electrodes differing in design but the most common is the clark-type electrode. It utilises a annular silver reference electrode (anode) and a glass coated platinum electrode (cathode) connected to a small external voltage source to charge the circuit with a potential difference of 500-700 mV. This is called polarising voltage. Oxygen gets reduced at the cathode giving rise to a current which is proportional t the concentration of oxygen in the solution provided that the polarising voltage remains approximately 700 mV. Oxygen from the solution diffuses in through a thin semi-permeable membrane which separates the electrodes from the test solution (Fig. 8.2). Both electrodes are immersed in the same solution of at saturated KCl.

The electroreduction of oxygen at the cathode which gives rise to current occurs according to the following equation.

$$O_2 + 2H_2O + 2e^- \longrightarrow H_2O_2 + 2OH + 2e^- \longrightarrow 2OH^-$$

$$OH^- + KCl \longrightarrow KOH + Cl^-$$

The electrons required for this electroreduction are produced at the reference electrode (anode) as follows:

$$4Ag^\circ + 4Cl^- \longrightarrow 4AgCl + 4e^-$$

The whole unit is mounted on a magnetic stirrer and a magnetic follower (flea) placed inside the reaction vessel. This keeps the test solution constantly stirred so as to obtain correct values of change in dissolved oxygen levels. Since the rate of dissolution of oxygen is temperature dependent, it is important to keep temperature constant. This is achieved by means of circulation of water in a water jacket around the reaction vessel.

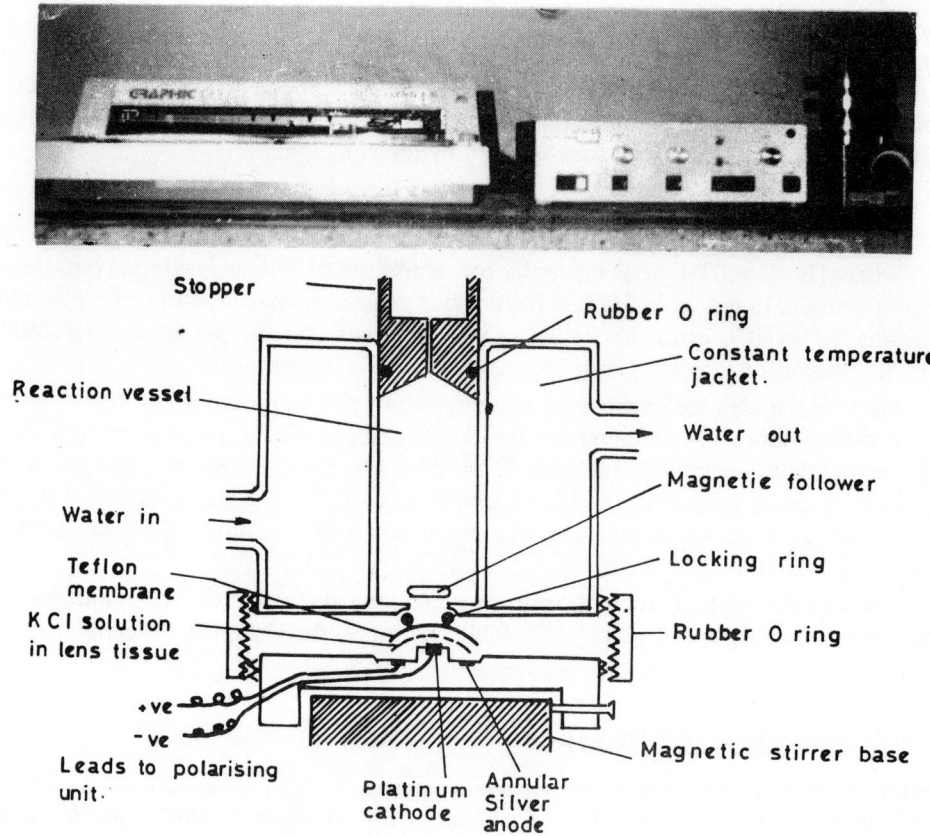

Fig. 8.2 : Diagram of a dismantled rank electrode. (Inset) The oxygen electrode (Right) with control Box (Centre) and graphic recorder (Left).

Both the water jacket and the reaction vessel are made of special type of transparent plastic so that photosynthetic studies requiring the use of light, can be carried out.

The unit is connected to a control box which takes electrical signals from the electrode and conveys it to a chart recorder.

The semi-permeable membrane used is generally teflon. This is highly permeable leading to quick establishment of equilibrium, but it responds differently for the same values of dissolved oxygen in gas and liquid. Less permeable membranes include polypropylene and polyethylene membranes which show little difference in response to liquid and gas.

Calibration of the Electrode

(1) Calibration is made with a liquid standard or gas standard which has been equilibrated with water vapour. Either standard must be equilibrated to the measuring temperature.

(2) The proper scale is selected certain instruments have more than one scale to accomodate wide ranges sometimes encountered during analysis.

(3) A standard usually distilled water is added to the reaction vessel, the magnetic follower introduced and the instrument is switched on for 30 minutes warm up time. During this time, the lid of the reaction vessel is kept open. The pen recorder stabilises at a particular point. This is taken as dissolved oxygen concentration of the standard whose value can be obtained from the following table.

Temperature (°C)	O_2(ppm)	O_2 (μMole/ml)
0	14.16	0.442
5	12.37	0.386
10	10.92	0.341
15	9.76	0.305
20	8.84	0.276
25	8.11	0.253
30	7.52	0.230
35	7.02	0.219

(4) If now a few crystals of sodium dithionite ($Na_2S_2O_4$) are added, all the oxygen is used up in accordance with the following reaction:

$$Na_2S_2O_4 + O_2 + H_2O \longrightarrow NaHSO_4 + NaHSO_3$$

The pen recorder moves a certain distance and stabilises at a particular point on the chart. This is the zero point of dissolved oxygen concentration. This point is adjusted with the zero calibration control of the recorder.

(5) This process is repeated several times till the zero concentration and standard concentration need no further adjustment.

(6) The number of divisions between the zero and standard correspond to the standard oxygen concentration. Hence, one division would represent a certain dissolved oxygen concentration e.g:

If 10 divisions = x μmol 1^{-1} oxygen

1 division = 0. x μmol 1^{-1} oxygen

(7) The instrument is thus calibrated and ready to determine unknowns.

3.1 Applications

The oxygen electrode is being put to increasingly wide uses because of easy portability of the instrument which is also inexpensive and does not require much expertise in handling.

Clinical Uses: Oxygen content of blood requires assessment during oxygen therapy. Oxygen electrodes have been designed to be small enough to be inserted into a blood vessel. However this involves the danger of infection or blood clot formation. Hence a transcutaneous electrode system has been devised to measure oxygen levels in the blood without having to pierce the skin. In this a small area on the skin, say earlobe or fingertip is heated externally to 43°C, and the electrode is held tightly to the depilated skin surface by an air-tight bond. A polypropylene membrane separates the heated skin surface from the electrode assembly, which consists of a polarised platinum cathode surrounded by a silver ring - type anode held at a constant temperature, usually 43°C. Oxygen in the blood diffuses from the blood capillary through the skin and electrode membrane and actuate the clark-type electrode to produce the reading.

Chloroplast and Mitochondrial Studies: Oxygen evolution in cyanobacteria, algae, chloroplasts ie those containing photosystem II can be studied using a suitably illuminated a Clark oxygen electrode. The oxygen content of the suspension medium is normally reduced below 100% oxygen by bubbling nitrogen through it so that oxygen produced stays in soltution and is recorded. Respiratory control studies and the effect of various inhibitors on mitochondrial respiration can also be studied using the oxygen electrode. Inhibitors of respiration slow down the rate of respiration.

Enzyme assays : Activity of enzymes which require oxygen for reaction eg. Glucose oxidase, catalase etc. can be studied using the Clark type oxygen electrode.

Microorganism studies: Bacteria which use oxygen as a terminal electron acceptor çan be studied using an oxygen electrode and the effect of electron inhibitors determined. The efficiency of different carbohydrates as respiratory substrates can be studied by comparing the rate of oxygen uptake.

9

TECHNIQUES WITH RADIOISOTOPES

1. ISOTOPES AND RADIOACTIVITY

Isotopes are different atoms of the same element having same atomic number but different atomic weights. The different atomic weights arise due to difference in the number of neutrons in the nucleus of the atom. e.g Hydrogen has three isotopes, normal hydrogen (H) having an atomic weight of 1.00814, deuterium (H) having an atomic weight of 2.01474 and tritium (H) having an atomic weight of 3.01701. All three have the same atomic number - 1. Tritium is radioactive. Radioactivity is a phenomenon in which nuclei of atoms of certain unstable isotopes decay or disintegrate spontaneously by releasing α-particles, β-particles or γ-rays. Such isotopes are called Radioisotopes.

α-particles are composed of two protons and two neutrons and thus are identical to Helium nuclei, He.

$$_{84}^{210}\text{Po} \longrightarrow _{82}^{206}\text{Pb} + _{2}^{4}\text{He (}\alpha\text{-particle)}$$

The particles move relatively slowly, but due to their mass they have a high momentum, travel in straight lines, not deflected from their path. Normally they are only deflected by direct collision with a nucleus.

β-articles are electrons released from the nucleus by decay of a neutron into a proton and an electron.

$$_{6}^{14}\text{C} \longrightarrow _{7}^{14}\text{N} + \beta\text{-particle}$$

Their energy spectrum depends on the speed with which the electron leaves the nucleus. β- particles are emitted from a given radioisotope over a continous range of energy upto a maximum value (E_{max}) which is characteristic of each radioisotope. They have little mass - about 1/7 400 the mass of α-particles. As it traverses material, it causes ionisation and excitation of orbital electrons. β- particles produced by ^{3}H and ^{14}C are weak with little penetrating power ('soft' β-particle) but those produced by ^{32}P are more energetic ('Hard' β- particles) and have greater penetrating power.

α-radiation is sometimes emitted during the course of radioactive decay if one of the intermediate stages in the decay sequence has too much energy to maintain stability. These are similar to X-rays except for their origin. α-rays are derived from events in the nucleus of an atom which X-rays are caused by excitation of orbital electrons; α-rays are emitted by specific radioisotopes at characteristic energies, generally ranging from 10 K e V to 3 KeV. Because α-ray have neither mass nor change they can travel great distances through matter though their ionising power is leser than that of β-particles.

The nucleus of an atom of a radioactive isotope has a certain probability, characteristic for that isotope that it will decay at any instant. The probability remains constant independent of chemical reactions the atom may undergo. It is also independent of temperature or other physical conditions. Because the probability is constant for all atoms of a given isotope in a specialised period of time a constant fraction of the nuclei will have decayed. The half-life $(T_{1/2})$ of an isotope is that period of time during which half the radioactive atoms originally present will have decayed. It is mathematically related to , the radioactivity decay constant, as follows:

$$T_{1/2} = \frac{0.693}{\lambda}$$

2. IONISATION EFFECTS

Because α-particles are relatively massive and doubly charged, when they pass close to another atom they may strip some orbital electrons from this atom producing positive ions. An α-particle with an energy of 1.5 Mev can produce about 2×10^5 positive ions in air before its energy is expended, β-particles also lead to ionisation of materials through which they pass. Being less massive, they travel faster and hence spend less time in the vicinity of other atoms and have less time to remove electrons from them. The ionisation effects caused by α- particles are therefore much less intense than those produced by β-particles. γ-rays being uncharged have no appreciable force fields, they do not lead directly to ionisation of materials. However they interact with mater in three unique ways indirectly producing energetic electrons.

(i) Low energy γ-radiation (< 0.5 MeV) can transfer all their energy to orbital electrons of atoms of the absorbing medium. The energy is thus transformed to the kinetic energy of the electrons which ejects out as the "Photoelectron".

(ii) Medium energy γ-radiation (0.5 - 1.0 MeV) may interact with electrons by inelastic collision and transfer only a portion of their energy in the process. The electron ejected (now termed Compton Electron) has lesser energy than the energy of the incident γ-radiation.

(iii) High energy γ-rays having energy more than 1.02 MeV react directly with the nucleus producing an electron - positron pair. This is a unique process in which high energy γ- rays are transformed into matter. The resulting positron reacts with the surrounding matter by colliding with an electron. The mass of both positron and electron are annihilated to become two 0.51 MeV photons.

Several devices for the measurement of radioactivity are based on the measurement of this ionisation in gas filled chambers. Gas ionisation detectors such as ion chambers, proportional counters, and Geiger - Mueller counters. Before considering any of the measurement techniques it makes sense to first make ourselves familiar with measurement units of radioactivity.

3. MEASUREMENT UNITS

Measurement units can be classified into three types.

(a) Unit of exposure of radioactivity i.e. the amount of radiation energy directed at a material. The most common unit is Rontgen (R) which is defined as the quantity of X - or γ-radiation which produces in air, ion of either sign carrying a charge of 2.58 x 10^{-4} C/Kg of air. Rontgen was restricted to radiations below 3 MeV. Because of the difficulty of measuring the ionisations in air of the very energetic secondary electrons, RAD was introduced.

(b) RAD or Radiation Absorbed Dose is the unit of absorbed radiation energy. It is defined as the absorption of 10^{-2} Joules of radiation energy per kg of material. The SI unit of absorbed dose is Gray (Gy) defined as 1J/Kg and therefore one hundred times larger than RAD. Since the energy absorbed in tissue corresponding to an exposure to one Rontgen is 0.0095 Joules/Kg one Rontgen gives an absorbed dose of 0.95 RAD.

(c) Unit of activity. This was until recently Curie (Ci) defined as the number of disintegrations per second (dps) occuring in 1 gram of pure Radium (^{226}Ra). It was arbitrarily fixed at 3.7 x 10^{10} dps.

i.e.

$$1 \text{ Ci} = 3.7 \times 10^{10} \text{ dps}$$

In SI, the Curie has been replaced by Becquerel (Bq). The two are related as:

$$2.703 \times 10^{-11} \quad \text{Ci} = 1 \text{ Bq}$$
$$3.7 \times 10^{10} \quad \text{Bq} = 1 \text{ Ci}$$

Specific activity is defined as the amount of radioactivity in a given weight of material and is usually expressed as Curies, disintegrations rate or count rate, per unit mass of element eg. the specific activity of C is 19 counts per minute per gram.

4. MEASUREMENT TECHNIQUES

Radioactivity is detected and calculated by measurements made by observing physical or chemical changes in appropriate device. The most common method is by measuring the amount of ionisation caused in air or other gases. Though this is the most important dosimetric method, there are many other systems of detection some of which are discussed below.

Scintillation detectors convert the radiation energy of ionising particles into pulses of light. The size of pulse is proportional to the energy deposited in the crystalline or liquid scintillant.

Some semi-cinductors show an altered conductivity during exposure to radiation. This method is similar to the ionisation chamber measurement except that the current is flowing in the solid semi-conductor crystals and not in the gas of the ionisation chamber.

In Ferrous sulphate dosimetry the $FeSO_4$ is converted to $Fe_2(SO_4)_3$ when irradiated. Chemical titrations with $K_2Cr_2O_7$ may be used to determine the amount of ferric ion and therefore radioactivity present.

Caloriemetry involves the measurement of rise in temperature produced by radiation in an insulated mass of unknown thermal capacity.

When LiF and many other crystals are heated after being exposed to radiation, they emit light; this is called thermoluminiscence. The absorption of radiation energy causes free electrons to be trapped in the lattice imperfections of the crystalline structure. These trapping levels lie between the valence band and the conduction band; the electrons can remain trapped for a considerable time. If the temperature of the crystal is raised, the electrons are excited from the trapping levels to the conduction band and then return to valence level with emission of light. Thermoluminiscence devices may be used as powders in capsules or sachets. Thermoluminiscent dosimeters are widespread in laboratories for personnel monitoring.

Photographic emulsions consist of AgX crystals or grains dispersed in gelatin. Radiation absorbed in an individual grain forms a latent image and the chemical action of development reduces the grain to silver. The blacker the film is, as measured by densitometry, the more dose it has received. This again is used for personnel protection, in the form of film badges.

Certain plastics and glasses become increasingly opaque with increasing radiation dose.

4.1 Scintillation Counting Systems

Scintillation counting is a means of detecting radiation via production of light flashes (scintillation). Energy of radiation is used to produce pulses of light which are counted. Substances called 'fluors' or scintillators fluoresce upon irradiation. The phenomenon of fluorescence has been discussed elsewhere and here it should suffice to say that fluorescence is emission of radiation of longer wavelength, as compared to wavelength of incident radiation. This many appear in the visible, region of the spectrum and energy is emitted as photons which are counted by associated electornic equipment (Fig. 9.1).

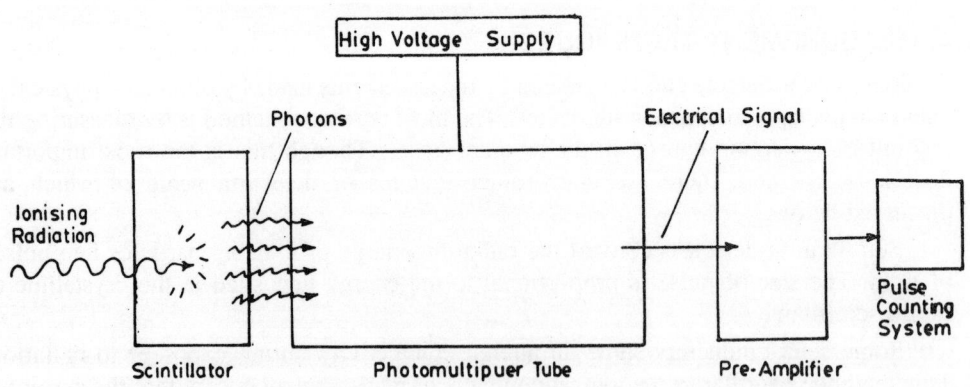

Fig. 9.1 : Simplified mechanism of scientilation counting.

The photomultiplier tube transforms the emitted photons into electrical signal, the magnitude of this signal is increased by more than a million times. In order that the multiplication is reproducible an extremely stable high voltage power must be supplied. The pre-amplifier further multiplies the photomultiplier output. This allows high counting rates to be achieved using scintillation counting.

The pulse height analyser differentiates among energies of the incident γ-rays. This analyser classifies pulses according to their height or amplitude. A single channel pulse height analyser consists of two variable discriminators which allow selection of lower and upper levels of detection. The lower discriminator setting is termed the base. The upper discriminator setting is selected by adding a voltage increment to the base. These two discriminators together with an anticoincidence circuit allow only those energies between the two discriminator levels to pass to the scaler. The scaler displays the counts accumulated during the counting period i.e it registers the number of pulses received.

Depending on whether the fluor is a solid or liquid there are two systems viz. solid scintillation counting and liquid scintillation counting. The fluor generally used for solid scintillation counting is a single large crystal of sodium iodide containing thallium as activator. The crystal surrounds the sample to increase counting efficiency. The sodium iodide crystals being hygroscopic (absorb water) in nature, are kept in light reflecting aluminium sachets which are completely closed except where attached to the photomultiplier tube through a transparent window.

Low energy β emitters like ^3H and ^{14}C cannot be counted by solid scintillation counting because the weak emissions cannot traverse the aluminium envelope of the scintillation crystals. This necessitates an intimate mixture of the isotope dissolved in liquid fluor so that there is no self absorption of β or α-particles and efficient energy transfer occurs. Liquid scintillation derives its name from the liquid mixture composed of isotope sample, fluor dissolved in an organic solvent. The mixture of organic solvent (usually toluene) and the fluor is often called "cocktail". For samples containing water, dioxane can be used as solvent. The fluors are generally complex heterocyclic, organic compounds which when excited emit photons in the near ultraviolet and visible regions. The fluors generally comprise less than 1% of the cocktail. Some organic fluors used are PPO (p- terphenyl, 2,5-diphenyloxazole) and POPOP (1,4-bis-2-(5-phenyloxazolyl)-benzene. PPO is the primary solute. POPOP is the secondary solute and is used to shift the fluorescence of PPO to longer wavelength for better matching to the spectral response of photomultiplier tubes. This procedure increases the counting yield and is generally used in measurement of H.

The emissions from the sample interact with the material surrounding them and cause excitation first of the solvent molecules. This excitation energy of solvent is transferred to the solute, the fluor, causing excitation of fluor electrons. The excited electrons in the fluor emit photons of light as they fall back to the ground state. These photons of light are detected by the photomultiplier tube and result in electrical pulses as in solid state counters (Fig. 9.2). Power supplies for high voltage and stable d.c. supply

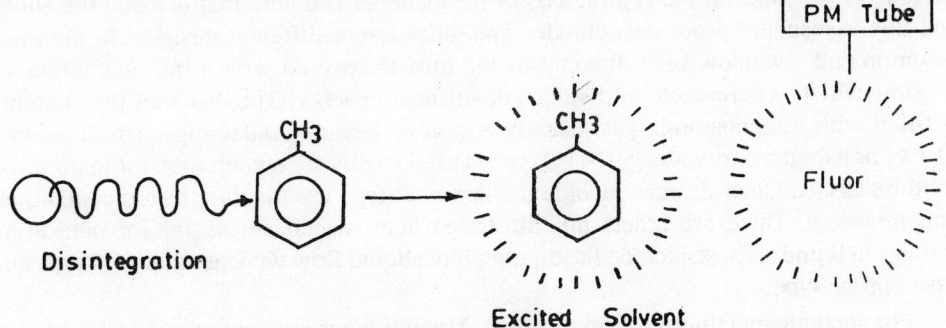

Fig. 9.2 : Liquid scintillation counting.

area same as those in solid state counters except that here, two potentials are supplied for paired photomultiplier tubes.

Since the low energy ranges of β-emissions result in photomultiplier output of the same magnitude as the thermionic emission coincidence circuitry has been used. This ensures that only pulses seen simultaneously (usually within less than 20 nanosecond) are registered. Pulses from the two detection circuits are passed through a coincidence circuit and electronically added up. Pulses then pass to two or more channels each consisting of a linear amplifier, pulse height analyser and scaler, as in solid state systems (Fig. 9.3)

Liquid scintillation counting though ideal for counting weak emissions, poses the problem of "Quenching". This is especially true of biological samples which may contain a great variety of chemical compounds. Even oxygen in the air and chemicals in the sample result in quenching. Quenching is of three types: chemical, chromatic and optical. Chemical quenching is caused by various polar absorb energy from excited solvent molecules, preventing, partly, the excitation of the fluor. Colour quenching can be expected whenever the fluor solution does not have its characteristic light blue colour due to impurities. Yellow and red solutions especially may·absorb the blue light which is emitted by the fluors. Optical quenching, results when the mixture of scintillation cocktail and sample result not in true solutions but in suspensions. Quenching decreases the detectable energy released by the isotopes. Hence it should be minimised. However, quenching is often unavoidable and the degree of quenching unpredictable. Therefore, it should be corrected for. Correction for quenching i.e. determination of efficiency (E) can be brought about by using the following relationship.

$$\% \, E \, = \, \frac{cpm}{dpm} \, \times 100$$

Disintegrations per minute (dpm) is an absolute number proportional to the isotopic content of sample while counts per minute (cpm) refers to the detected counts which is always less than dpm due to quenching.

4.2 Geiger - Mueller Counter

The Geiger - Mueller counter utilises the ionisations produced in air or gas by radioactive disintegrations.

The electrical signal is produced by a special tube (Fig.9.4). The tube consists of a chamber, the inner surface being coated with an electrical conductor, and this is made the cathode of the tube. At the central axis of the chamber is a wire that is made the anode and this is insulated from the cathode. The tubes are of different designs. In the most common end - window tube, the end of the tube is covered with a thin membrane or window which is permeable to particles of sufficient energy. The inside of the chamber is filled with a monoatomic gas, usually Argon or Helium containing a small amount (0.1%) or halogen or organic gas. This type is used mostly for quantitative estimations on solid materials. Other designs include the thin wall type used mainly inside contamination monitors. There are others not illustrated here, which are useful for measuring activity in liquids. These include the dipping type, liquid flow type, annular well type and tissue probe type.

For accurate quantitative work Geiger - Mueller tubes are contained in a lead block which also surrounds the sample chamber to shield the tube and chamber from outside radiations which give rise to counts in the apparatus when no sample is present.

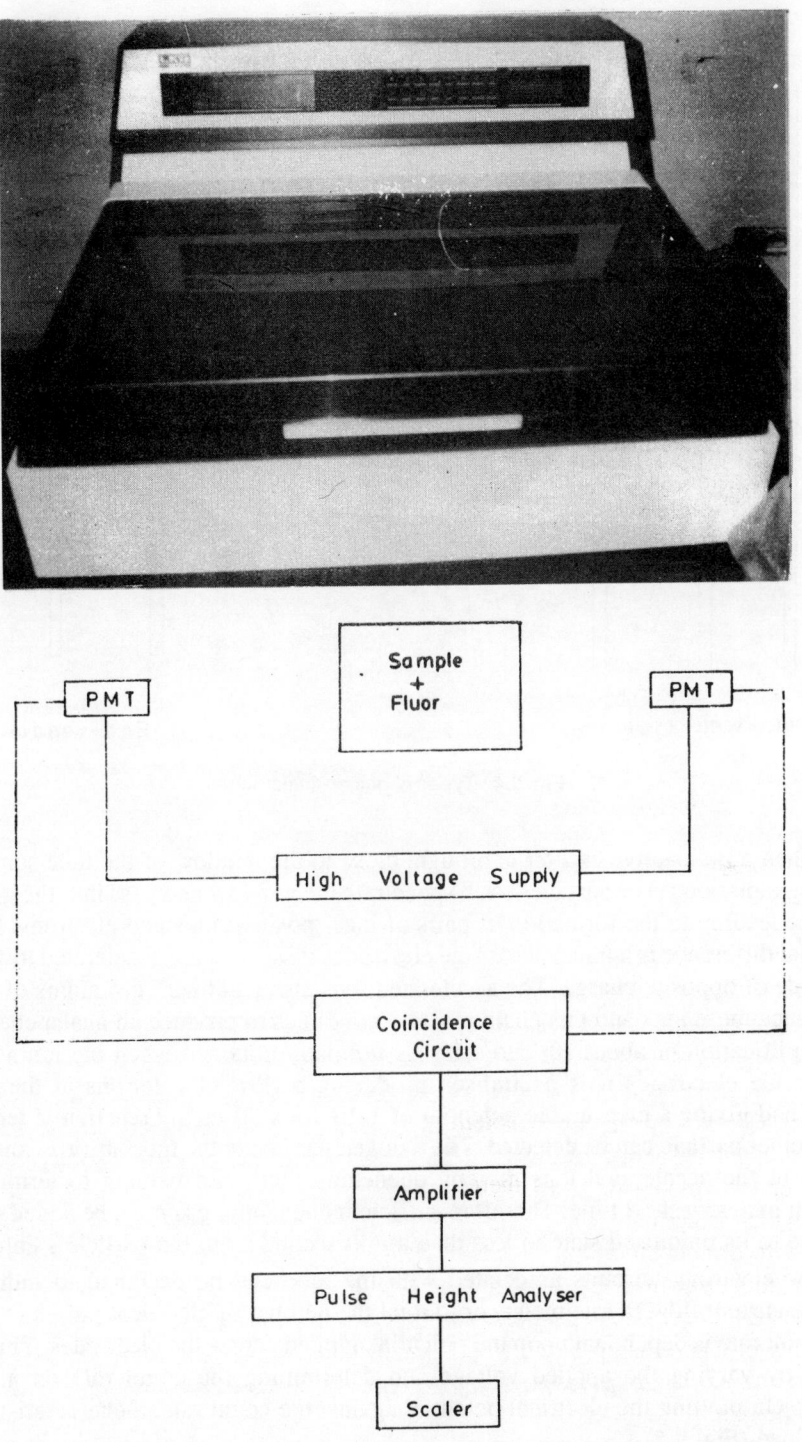

Fig. 9.3 : Block diagram of a liquid scintillation counter (Inset) A liquid scintillation counter.

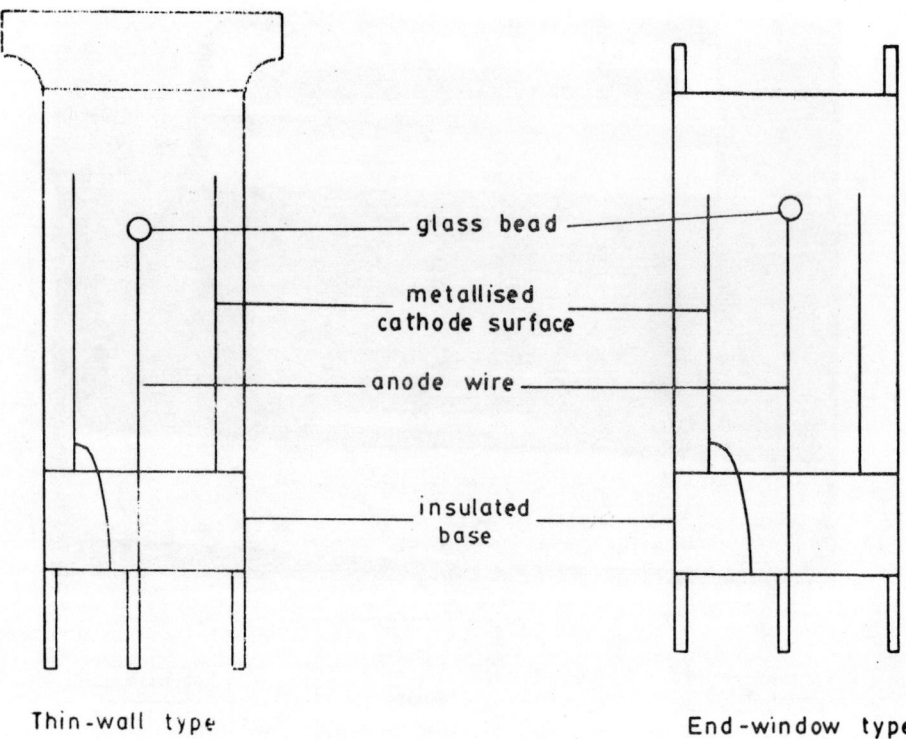

Fig. 9.4 : Types of geiger-muller tubes.

When a radioactive emitter is brought close to the window of the tube some of the ionising radiation (γ) or particles (α, β) penetrate the window and pass into the gas inside the tube leading to the formation of pairs of ions- positive ions and electrons. If a high potential difference is applied across the electrodes these ions are accelerated towards the electrode of opposite charge. The accelerated ions also react with gas atoms of the tube to produce more ions and this chain reaction continues to produce an avalanche of ions. An amplification of about 10^6 to 10^8 is normally obtained when the ion avalanche reaches the electrodes it is neutralised producing a flow of electrons in the external circuit and giving a measurable potential of 1-10 volts. Thus the reaction is terminated and another particle can be detected. The halogen gas inside the tube absorbs some of the energy of the accelerated ions thereby quenching them and helping to terminate the reaction in a very short time. Therefore sufficient quenching gas must be added to return the tube to its unionised state in less than a millisecond from the particle's entry.

The electronic circuits associated with the tube can be designed to indicate the average current flow (a rate meter) or to total the number of electrical pulses (a scaler). The count rate is dependent upon the potential applied across the electrodes. This can be shown by varying the applied voltage and determining the count rate on a suitable sample. On plotting the electrical potential against the count rate, a characteristic curve is obtained (Fig. 9.5).

At low voltage the curve is exponential and slight changes in voltage cause considerable changes in the count rate. At higher voltages the curve becomes linear over this

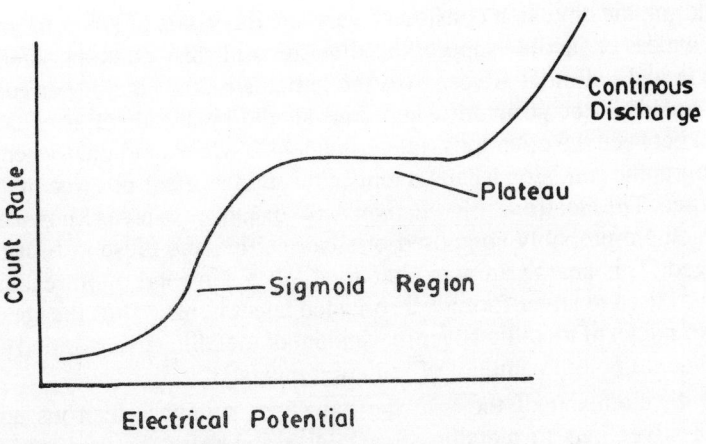

Fig. 9.5 : Charecteristic sigmoid curve.

region; the voltage across electrodes a great enough to cause particles to move sufficiently fast to produce maximum ionisation of the tube gas. At even higher voltages the count rate increases exponentially as the Geiger tube goes into continuous discharge, the voltage being great enough to break down the insulating properties of the gas inside the tube. For maximum stability the tube is operated in the plateau region where changes in voltages have little effect upon count rate. In the plateau region the tube is operating at near its maximum efficiency and therefore no distinction can be made between particles of differing energy content providing of course, that the particles have sufficient energy to penetrate the tube window. This method of counting is therefore an all or nothing process. As in the case of scintillation counters, the efficiency of the tube is cpm/dpm x 100.

When energy of radiation is low as from ^3H particles, most of the particles are absorbed either before they reach the Geiger tube of the counter or by the window material. Hence tritium cannot be counted on this type of system unless special windowless gas flow tubes are used.

The conditions under which a Geiger Mueller tube is usually operated is such that the tube gas is almost totally ionised and hence electrical pulse size is not influenced by the nature of the incident radiation. However, at low voltages α and β-particles produce different degrees of ionisation and different intensities of signal. Consequently by the use of suitable discriminator circuits either in a normal Geiger system or in a low voltage ionisation chamber α, β particles from same or different sources can be detected. This type of counting is termed proportional counting since the size of the signal is proportional to the amount of ionisation produced by the incident radiation and hence varies with the nature of this radiation.

4.3 Autoradiography

Autoradiography is the detection of radioactivity using photographic emulsions. This is a techique by which radioactivity can only be detected and not measured. However, this factor does not in any way lessen its importance as a unique technique in biology. In conjunction with several other techniques, autoradiography is widely used in molecular biology, we shall briefly aquaint ourselves with some of these techniques, later in the chapter.

A photographic emulsion consists of very small crystals of silver bromide in gelatin mounted n a glass or flexible support the silver bromide also contains small quantities of silver sulfide and colloidal silver. Also the lattice structure is not perfect but contains spaces or "holes" in the structure where ions should be and there are silver ions out of place and in between the other ions (interstitial ions). When a radioactive emission passes into a photographic emulsion it causes ionisation and sets electrons free in the ionic silver bromide lattice. The electrons migrate over short distances to areas known as "sensitivity specks" which are probably composed of silver sulfide and these in turn become negatively charged. This charge attracts interstitial silver ions and upon reaching the speck they are neutralised to silver forming a so-called latent image. Thus the specks act as loci for growth of nuclei of metallic silver the amount of metallic silver formed at these points being dependent upon the amount of radiation received.

During development of the film the developer supplies electrons and causes the reduction of silver ions to metallic silver atoms and these are responsible for visible image. However, because of the catalytic effect of the metallic atoms already produced by the radiation the silver ions in the region of the latent image are reduced by the developer very much faster than those regions where there is no latent image. Hence, if development is correctly timed only the former produce a visible image and this image will reflect the sites of exposure of the emulsion to radiation. Thiosulfate present in the fixer solution removes unexpected silver bromide and hence stabilises the image.

5. COUNTING STATISTICS

If a single radioactive sample is counted several times under identical conditions and the count rate is corrected for radioactive decay or else the decay correction is negligible, the individual count rates will be observed to deviate about a mean value. These deviations are due to random nature of radioactive decay. The understanding of these statistical effects is necessary in the consideration of experimental design and in the interpretation of experimental results. Counting statistics follow closely the Poisson probability distribution. By a special property of the Poisson distribution the standar deviation (D) of a registered number of counts c is equal to the square root of that number for c registered counts.

$$D = \sqrt{c}$$

...... (1)

The standard deviation increases as the square root of the number of counts but decreases as a percentage of the counts. If in equation (1) both sides are divided by the period of counting t, the result is the standard deviation of the count rate r

$$\frac{D}{t} = \frac{\sqrt{c}}{t} = Dr$$

since $c = r t$

$$Dr = \frac{\sqrt{r t}}{t}$$

The number of counts c collected in any counting interval are due to true counts of the sample plus those due to background. There is significant background radiation in almost any location. This is due to cosmic rays, cosmic ray - induced activity such as ^{14}C and to naturally occuring radioactive materials in the earth's crust eg. ^{226}Ra, ^{232}Th and ^{40}K. The latter all have associated γ-rays. The cosmic ray contribution varies with altitude and the composition of the earth's crust varies with location. All radiation detector counter systems have an associated background counting rate due to above sources and also electronic noise. The background count rate is commonly reduced by shielding or by special electronic circuitry. The background radiation will be a function of the type of detector shielding, location, discriminator settings etc.

The variations of background are independent of the variations of the sample activity and the appropriate error terms add as the sum of the squares. Therefore Variance (D^2) due to sample activity alone is

$$D_s^2 = D_{s+b}^2 + {}_bD^2$$

where

D_s^2 = Variance due to sample alone

D_{s+b}^2 = Variance due to count of sample + background

D_b^2 = Variance due to background

For a total of C accumulated counts due to sample and background counts the standard deviation of the sample count is given by

$$D_s = \sqrt{C_{s+b}} + C_b$$

where,

C_{s+b} = Total counts due to sample + background

C_b = Total counts due to background counted alone.

If t_s = Counting time for sample in the presence of background

t_b = Counting time for background

Then the standard deviation of sample counting rate Dr_s,

$$Dr_s = \frac{r_{s+b}}{t_s} + \frac{r_b}{t_b}$$

In tracer experiments, discussed below, the net counting rate of samples very commonly approaches, or is even less than background counting rates. In order to choose the best division of time for counting sample and for counting background to obtain the minimum error, the following may be used,

$$\frac{t_b}{t_s} = \frac{r_b}{r_{s+b}}$$

6. BIOLOGICAL USES OF RADIOISOTOPES

Radioisotopes are widely used to study physiological processes of biology. A small quantity of radioisotope called Tracer or label is introduced into the system to be studied and its behavior is observed by tracing the position of the radioisotope within the system. The substance to be traced is called Tracee. The label is incorporated into the tracee through biological growth, chemical synthesis or exchange processes.

The usefulness of radioisotopes in biological studies stems largely from the fact that the rate of radioactive decay is independent of physical or chemical conditions and so the rate of decay of ^{32}P in for example PO of ATP and DNA will be constant. Also, the methods used to count isotopes are extremely sensitive and therefore very small quantities (called labels) can be detected in large quantities of unlabelled material. An activity of as little as 10^{-3} to 10^{-10} uries can be detected by ordinary equipment although the quantity of material corresponding to this activity depends upon the specific activity of the sample and the quantity of radioactive material on the half life of the isotope. This considerable sensitivity of detection enables the use of very small amounts of radioactive material making such experiments economical. At the same time in the case of physiological experiments where the normal metabolic balance could easily be upset by unnaturally high concentration of materials added merely to facilitate detection. Detection and estimation of isotopes by monitoring their radiation also has the advantage that the sample is not always destroyed or altered and may be retained for further study. Since radioactive and non-radioactive samples of the same compound are chemically equivalent, small amounts of labelled compounds become intimately mixed with much larger quantities of unlabelled material in the organism and cannot be distinguished from it except for their radioactivity. Therefore isotopically labelled compounds can be detected in the presence of pre- =existing unlabelled material and this is of great significance in many studies.

In biological investigations, isotopes which emit particles are not normally used as tracers because they belong to elements of high atomic number that is above 82. Such elements are rarely important metabolically though some uptake studies have been made. The most important isotopes in biological studies are isotopes of those elements which are found in living systems. These include ^{3}H, ^{14}C, ^{32}P ^{35}S and ^{36}Cl which are emitters. A number of isotopes with some biological significance emit radiation and perhaps **the** most often used are ^{59}Fe, ^{24}Na, ^{125}I and ^{131}I. These light isotopes are rarely found naturally and have to be produced artificially principally by one of the three types of reactions.

(i) Bombardment with a neutron and elimination of radiation.

$$^{23}_{11}\text{Na} + \,^{1}_{c}\text{n} \longrightarrow \,^{24}_{11}\text{Na} + \gamma$$

(2) Bombardment with a neutron and elimination of a proton

$$^{32}_{16}\text{S} + \,^{1}_{0}\text{n} \longrightarrow \,^{32}_{15}\text{P} + \,\text{p}$$

(3) Bombardment with a neutron and elimination of an particle

$$^{27}_{13}\text{Al} + \,^{1}_{0}\text{n} \longrightarrow \,^{24}_{11}\text{Na} + \,^{4}_{2}\text{He}$$

The criteria of an ideal tracer is that it should be indistinguishable from the tracee at the unit level, the introduction of the tracer should not disturb the system, the half life should be long enough to last through the course of the experiment, it should be easy to incorporate as well as easy to detect in the system.

6.1 Tracer Dilution Technique

The tracer dilution technique introduced by Hevesey is particularly useful when quantitative separations are not possible or are too tedious for the systems under study. If a radioactive specimen of one of the compounds present in the mixture is added to the mixture, the label becomes uniformly distributed throughout the mixture. When the compound is reisolated some of the label will be present and hence can be counted and the specific activity of the sample calculated. The concentration of the non-radioactive compound in the mixture can be determined from the extent to which it has diluted the radioactive additive i.e., weight of unlabelled material

$$= \text{weight labelled} \quad \frac{\text{specific activity additive}}{\text{specific activity isolate}} - 1$$

It is not necessary to isolate all material under study from the mixture because the label will be uniformly diluted in it. It is however, necessary to purify the extract rigorously to remove any radioactive contaminants. A variation of the tracer dilution technique called "inverse tracer dilution" enables determination of the amount of tracer in a system by the addition of a known amount of tracee.

6.2 Radioimmunoassay (RIA)

Radioimmunoassay is one of the most important techniques in the clinical and biochemical fields for quantitative analysis of steroids hormones, drugs and are specially useful for testing the sera from immunised animals for antibody response and for screening hybridomas for secretion of specific antibody Immunoassays are very sensitive and specific and therefore are commonly used for a great variety of measuremtns both in research and analytical laboratories. Several refinements of the basic technology have been developed. The most common techniques use a radioactively labelled antigen or antibody and involves competition for antibody binding between labelled and unlabelled antigens. The technique is based on the competition between unlabelled antigen and a finite amount of the corresponding radiolabelled antigen for a limited number of antibody binding sites in a fixed amount of antiserum. At equilibrium (with excess antigen) there will be both free antigen and antigen bound to the antibody. Under standard conditions the amount of labelled antigen bound to antibody will decrease as the amount of unlabelled antigen in the sample increases.

4 Ag* + 4 Ab   4 Ag*Ab

4 Ag + 4 Ag* + 4Ab   2Ag* Ab + 2Ag Ab + 2Ag + 2 Ag*

12 Ag + 4 Ag* + 4Ab Ag   Ab + 3Ag* Ab + 3Ag* + 9 Ag

where Ab, Ag, Ag* and AgAb are antibody, unlabelled antigen, labelled antigen and antibody antigen complex respectively.

By using known amounts of unlabelled antigen and a fixed amount of antibody and labelled antigen, the amount of labelled antigen bound as a function of the total antigen added is measured and a calibration curve constructed (Fig. 9.6).

This calibration curve may then be used to determine the amount of antigen in samples treated similarly.

Radioimmunoassays offer the following potential advantages.

(1) Sensitivity

(2) Simplicity

(3) Specificity

(4) The ability to measure any compound that is immunogenic confers on the technique the advantage of universal application.

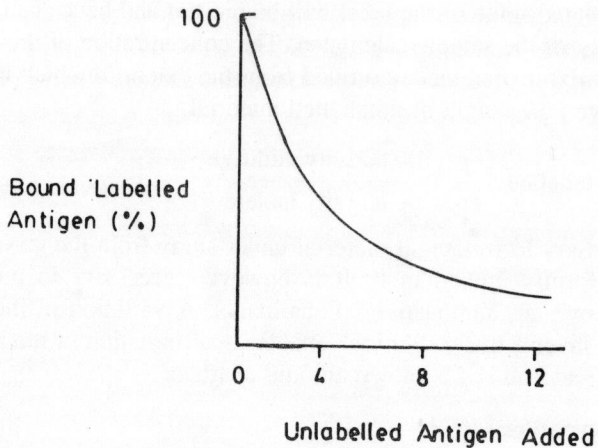

Fig. 9.6 : Calibration curve.

In spite of these, it is not free from drawbacks which include high costs of instruments used for measuring radioactivity and also the dangers involved in handling radioactive compounds. Hence alternative labels such as enzymes (ELISA - Enzyme Linked Immunosorbent Assay) or fluorochromes (fluorescence immuno-assay) have been used.

6.3 Miscellaneous Uses of Radioisotopes

It is often left to the researcher's imagination, the number of ways in which he can use a particular technique. On e such enterprising scientist has been Southern after whom the technique of Southern blotting is named. Molecular biology involves analysis of DNA in many ways. Electrophoresis of DNA results in the separation of DNA according to size. Now, it is often required to detect whether the required DNA piece is present or not. This can be achieved by transferring the DNA from the intact gel onto a piece of nitrocellulose paper placed in contact with it, using denaturation conditions, so that the DNA becomes bound to the paper in exactly the same pattern as that originally on the gel. This transfer called Southern blot can be achieved electrophoretically, or by drawing large volumes of buffer through both gel and paper. DNA thus transferred can now be treated with radiolabelled DNA molecule acting as "probe" to discover which bands of DNA contain sequences complementary to the probe after autoradiography of the paper.

The use of radiolabelled DNA probes together with subsequent autoradiography has been put to practice in many molecular biology techniques such as colony hybridisation to detect and locate mutant colonies of microorganisms growing on a Petri plate.

10

THE PERSONAL COMPUTER

1. INTRODUCTION

A computer which is used by one individual at a time and which does not require the support of other individuals to be operated is called a 'personal' computer.

Like all computer systems, the personal computer has a Hardware and Software. Hardware is the physical part of the machine while software is the more intangible stored program. Hardware includes the System Unit, Disk Drives, Display, Keyboard, Printer and other peripherals.

2. HARDWARE

The System Unit: The system unit is the heart and brain of the PC. It also includes the memory of the computer in RAM and ROM. RAM (Random Access Memory) is used to hold programs typed in by the user. This can have information written into it and retrieved from it. This is not permanent and is lost when the computer is turned off. The ROM (Read Only Memory) is used to store permanent programs. The programs stored in ROM cannot be altered by the user. These include programs which tell the computer how to accept information from the keyboard, programs to allow the user to store inforamtion in memory and modify it, programs to display the stored information and so on.

The processor performs all the operations and calculations and controls the activities of the entire system. The data and instructions are made available to the computer system on the Disk Drives. From the Disk Drives it is loaded onto the memory of the computer so that the processor can manipulate it as required.

Disk and Disk Drives: Application software or software that comes prepared to perform a specific type of task is usually kept on a Disk. The Disk, also called a Floppy can store data and information which made available to the computer system when required through Disk Drives. Hard Disks are faster and store much more information than Flexible Disks or Floppies. But they are disadvantageous since they cannot be removed and replaced. Hence Hard Disks are used till they are full, then their contents if needed are copied onto flexible Disks and the Hard Disk reused. Thus two Disk Drives including at least one flexible Disk Drive provide the advantage of being able to easily make copies for back-up.

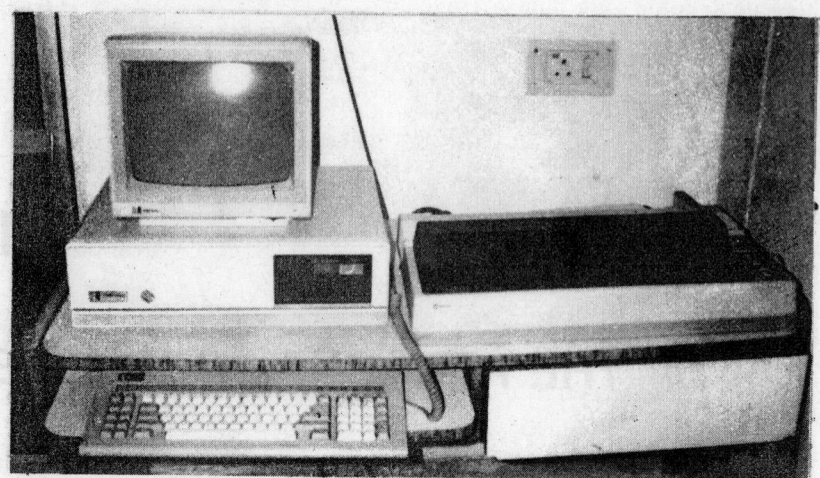

Fig. 10.1

The Keyboard: is an input device or a means to communicate with the Computer System. It looks like a type-writer with a few extra keys. Instructions can be given to the PC by simply pressing keys. What is typed appears on the 'TV like' unit called the Display.

The Display: The Display is known by many different names such as the Monitor, Console, Cathode Ray Tube (CRT), Visual Display Unit (VDU), Terminal, Screen. Whatever is entered via the keyboard first appears on the Display as also the PC's response, thus making it a very interactive device.

Printers: Printers are output devices which may be aded to the PC to obtain paper printouts of results.

3. SOFTWARE

There are two types of software. Systems Software and Applications Software. The systems software provides general capabilities to control the computer Hardware and peripherals, used facilities. The most important type of systems software is the operating system or O/S which consists of programs to manage the overall operation of the Computer System e.g. MS-DOS (Microsoft, Disk operating System) which gives the PC compatibility with other software.

Applications software are tailored specifically to particular tasks e.g. Finance, According, Data Base Management, Inventory Word Processing Computer Aided design etc. These can easily be used by persons who are not familiar with computer programming. Applications software includes programs which ask for data and type of output required. All this is typed in and in the no time the required output is displayed on the VDU. The output may be a histogram, a pie chart, a graph etc.

All software is a kind of Computer language that can be used to program a computer. There are many different languages. The most basic of these is machine language, a collection of very detailed, cryptic instructions that control the computer's internal circuitry. This is the natural dialect of the computer. However, machine languages are cumbersome to work with and hence some high level language is used, this instruction set is more compatible with human languages hence often called user - friendly languages. These include :

BASIC - Beginner's All Purpose Symbolic Instruction Code

Pascal - named after a French Scientist

FORTRAN - Formula Translation

COBOL - Commercial, Business Oriented Language

With the advent of personal computers, program packages were made available on floppy disks. A PACKAGE is computer jargon for a program or a set of programs which will run generally on a range of computers. These include among others.

WORDSTAR This package is, like all good packages, is user friendly and is guided by a series of menus. The usual sequence needed to use wordstar is first to load the wordstar disk into the main drive of computer then carry out the start-up procedure which differs from computer to computer. After this "boot up" procedure a prompt in the form of a letter A and > character appear on the left hand side of the screen. At that point the computer is usually awaiting a command as indicated by a bright rectangle called CURSOR immediately after the > character. In order to obtain Wordstar. WS followed by return is typed in and the opening menu is displayed on the screen. The only keys which will cause wordstar to do anything are those listed in the menu L F H D N P E O Y R X M or S. Press any other key and nothing will happen. Now press 'O' and the onscreen menu will be displayed. This will further tell about the keys to be pressed for particular commands. For example to print in italics, to print in bold letters, superscripts, subscripts etc. Thus, the use of wordstar enables one to produce an error - free text with the minimum of effort and without lengthy retyping of the text every time a change has to be made. The control keys instruct wordstar to perform certain operations on the text.

LOTUS - 123 : This is an electronic spreadsheet package. A spreadsheet is usually designed to eliminate the tedious process of having to work out complicated calculations over and over again manually, to allow storage and retrieval of data in an orderly manner and to allow graphical representation of statistics almost instantaneously among other things. Its greatest strength lies perhaps in its ability to instantly re-calculate every formula in the worksheet as and when required. A spreadsheet may be considered to be a large matrix with some data in each cell of the matrix. LOTUS-123 Spreadsheet, graphics and database serve as powerful tools for solving planning, finance and other problems.

123 graphics is particularly useful in research for storage and analyses of experimental data. 123 graphics can generate line, bar and pie graphs to help analyse data and illustrate results, highlighting significant variances, if any. A graph is any day worth a thousand numbers.

4. COMPUTER APPLICATIONS

The advent of computers has meant that calculations which were previously beyond contemplation because of time and drudgery involved in carrying them out, have now become possible. This has greatly expanded and accelerated research.

Computers also play an important role in present day hospital administration and in medical diagnostics, bio-analysis and therapeutic aspects in addition to controlling processing and evaluation of medical data.

4.1 Medical Diagnostics

(a) *CAT SCAN* Just as the discovery of X-rays in 1895 proved to be invaluable in medical diagnostics, the introduction of Computerised Axial Tomography (CAT) or Computerised Tomography (CT) is a resolutionary diagnostic tool, first introduced by Dr. Godfrey Hounsfield in 1969. This latest diagnostic aid helps in

- Speedy and sure diagnosis
- Eliminates the need for painful risky surgery for exploration and location of lesion or disease. It is life saving in accident cases where it can diagnose blood clots which can be evacuated immediately.
- Pin - pointing pathological spots resulting in accurate surgery. By coupling standard CT equipment with the computer graphics used to design the F-15 and other aircraft, three dimensional screen images of a patient's skull can be generated and manipulated to show the surgeons what they need to do - even what the results of their surgery will be - before they ever pick up a scalpel.

In this technique, the patient is made to lie down and a narrow X-ray beam is made to pass through the part of the body being scanned. When an X-ray beam passes through a tissue, it undergoes a change in intensity. This change or "attenuation" of intensity of X-ray beam depends on the atomic number and density of tissues it passes through and is detected by a crystal detector placed so as to receive the emerging X-ray beam. The crystal detector is optically coupled to a photomultiplier tube.

Several readings are taken at different angles by the detectors and fed into a computer which analyses all these attenuation values and reconstructs an image on the screen. The computer also stores data from which one can reconstruct slices in other planes thus helping to determine the exact position of the disease or lesion.

Apart from location of exact position of surgery, CT scanning also helps to PLAN surgery. For example, a young girl whose face was fractured across its entire width, in an automobile accident had two operations but her face was still distorted. Then the computer showed where a graft could go to remove the distortion and it worked.

(b) *NUCLEAR MEDICINE* The technology of nuclear medicine permits direct measurements to be made of body processes. Such study often produces large amounts of data, often in the form of quantities of radioactivity distributed is specific sites within the body, often changing over a period of time. The instrumentation utilised presents data either as quantities that can be plotted or analysed or as image analogs that allow the clinician to visualize the distribution of radioactive tracer materials within an organ or lesion. The full diagnostic potential of nuclear data cannot be realised without the aid of a computer.

The patient is given a tracer dose of a suitable isotope either orally or intravenously. The patient is then made to lie down and information gathering begins with the detector which moves around the body of the patient. Gamma rays emitted by the isotope are picked up by the lead collimator which is the focussing element of the camera. Each scintillation in the camera's detector crystal are read by photomultiplier tubes and fed out in voltage analogs that describe its intensity and spatial position with respect to X and Y co-ordinates. The camera's output is monitored directly on a cathode ray tube display. At the same time it may be fed into the computer memory system or onto disk storage. The voltage analog output from the camera is translated in the processing unit into the digital language of the computer through an in-built analog to digital converter.

The uses to which this data can be put depends on the imagination and programming skills of the operator. For example, the computer can be asked to quantify, combine. select, compare and display its answers either in the form of a graph, tables or images. The computer can also be directed to "add images", thus adding all counts, accumulated in a site over a specified time, for example, where the site first became visible against its background. This combines the identification of a site of interest with its intensification. Such versatility in processing data has made it possible to obtain very reliable diagnostic results.

4.2 Research

Computer technology can be used significantly in several research requirements.

(a) Statistics: Large amounts of data often need to be tabulated or analysed for various values for example χ values, standard deviation etc. These require repetitive procedures and calculations which can be performed very quickly and efficiently by computers. Statistical procedures are essential in biology particularly to test cause and effect systems of environmental and heriditary causes of diseases as well as studies on normal population groups.

(b) Simulation: In order to develop a better understanding of biological processes computer - based models can be built. Significant models have been constructed in areas of respiratory behavior, cardiac cycle Models of cell life - cycles give guidance to sequential radiation treatments in Cancer therapy.

(c) Graphics: Graphic representation of computer - produced results is required frequently to display data obtained from experiments. Graphics can also be used for investigation of biological processes. For example, valuable insights concerning embryonic evolution of the nervous system are being derived from graphically supported 3-D reconstructions from microscopic serial sections. Mechanics of limb motion can also be studied in a similar manner.

(d) Data collection: A large number of instruments used in modern research are computerised so as to provide the information obtained from the instrument in the required form. For example in spectrophotometers the change of absorbance of the sample at different wavelengths can be obtained in the form of a graph so that the peaks of the curves are noticeably clear and the λ_{max} of the sample can be easily read off this graph.

4.3 Drug Designing

Drugs work by binding to specific receptors (such as enzymes, DNA molecules, or proteins in the membrane of a cell) and triggering of the desired effect. The computer with its graphics and calculations can facilitate the understanding of this union by diagramming the receptor and the drug molecule that will fit it. The computer systems that are doing "molecular mapping" today rapidly digest incredibly large amount of information and then use it to build a visual model of a drug or chemical. A computer can display the molecular structure of any drug from a listing of thousands contained in its memory. By looking at and analysing one of these stored models, chemists can tell if a drug's particular arrangement of atoms is the molecular "key" that fits into and opens a biological "lock" (the receptor) within the body - perhaps to lower blood pressure, to prevent a pain signal from reaching the brain or to kill an invading bacterium.

When a chemist wants to know why different looking drugs act on the same receptor, he can ask the computer to superimpose them all on the screen so he can see how their atoms match up. For example, in a study to see how 4 chemicals act like dopamine, a natural substance in the body that helps transmit nerve signals (Parkinson's disease is associated with a lack of dopamine) it was found after all 4 chemicals merged on the screen, that all 4 had a ring of carbon atoms in the same location, common to each other. It seemed logical to assume that those atoms were at least part of the electronic key that opens the receptor's door and a clue to understanding of dopamine related diseases.

Thus computers are no longer mathematically biased. Biology has equally to take, if not more from computers.

INDEX